The Breast

Also by Oliver Cope, M.D.

Man, Mind and Medicine: The Doctor's Education
(Lippincott, 1968)

*Management of the Cocoanut Grove Burns at the
Massachusetts General Hospital* (editor)
(Lippincott, 1943)

The Breast

Its Problems—Benign and Malignant—
And How to Deal with Them

Oliver Cope, M.D.

Houghton Mifflin Company

Boston

The author is grateful for permission to reprint from "Laetrile: focus on the facts," by R. C. Eyerly, which appeared in *Ca — A Cancer Journal for Clinicians*, published by the American Cancer Society, and from a booklet entitled "Breast Problems in Women," published by the American College of Obstetricians and Gynecologists.

Library of Congress Cataloging in Publication Data

Cope, Oliver, date
    The breast : its problems, benign and malignant,
    and how to deal with them.
    Bibliography: p.
    Includes index.
    1. Breast—Tumors. I. Title. [DNLM: 1. Breast
neoplasms—Therapy. WP870 C782b]
RC280.B8C65   616.9'94'49   77-9045
ISBN 0-395-25709-3

Printed in the United States of America

V 10 9 8 7 6 5 4 3

To my Alice and our children

Contents

The Breast

Chapter 1

Why This Book?

CANCER OF THE BREAST has become a prime issue of health. New treatments have appeared and there is confusion regarding which to use — the old or the new. It is a time of rapid change, full of conflicting advice that is difficult even for a doctor to find his way through. The situation will be helped if patients as well as doctors are fully informed.

Until yesterday, the standard treatment for cancer of the breast was radical mastectomy. Today we realize that this surgical procedure cures only those patients whose cancer is confined to the breast and breast region. These are but one quarter of the patients; in three-quarters we now know that the cancer cells have escaped from the breast and spread to distant parts of the body before the operation was performed. These patients, despite hormonal and other treatments, have eventually died of the cancer. This knowledge explains why the mortality from cancer of the breast has not been significantly reduced in the last thirty years.

New knowledge, new modes of treatment have come from fields other than surgery. The cancer within the breast can be treated by irradiation without sacrificing the breast and, equally important, the spread of the cancer throughout the body can in many patients be stemmed by drugs. The outlook for both the quality and length of life has improved.

Cancer of the breast is a dread disease. If skin cancers are excluded, it is the most common cancer of women. It is not as common, however, as the recent publicity from the American Cancer Society and the National Cancer Institute would seem to imply. Only 7 percent of women in the United States are afflicted, which means that 93 percent of women never get it.[1,2,3] And, what is more, breast cancer is not on the increase. Its incidence has not changed significantly since 1939.

It arouses women's fears because it carries such a high mortality and its treatment has been so disfiguring. The fear is compounded because lumps of the breast are commonplace in a woman's life. Most of her lumps are benign, but the presence of a lump arouses the fear of cancer, and it is sometimes difficult even for the doctor to distinguish between the benign and cancerous lumps. If women are properly informed about the various types of lumps, how they occur, at what phases in their lives they are found, if they come to understand the relation of their menstrual cycles to the everyday lumpiness, they will be relieved of much of their anxiety. Physicians also will be helped by better understanding.

The development of the operation of radical mastectomy at the end of the nineteenth century improved the lot of women suffering from cancer of the breast. Large, painful, ulcerating tumors of the breast were eliminated. But the loss of the breast has proved a hardship, as devastating to some women as loss of the penis is to men.

When the only treatment was surgical removal of the breast, doctors had to turn their backs on the psychologically distressing aspects. With the arrival of alternative and less mutilating treatments, it is now time for women to assert their wishes, and for doctors to be more considerate in their choice of therapies.

Why am I writing this book for the general public? A look at what is going on today will make the reasons plain.

Medicine moves slowly. Doctors are loath to abandon a treatment with which they are familiar for a new one based on concepts seemingly untried. Usually the battles that bring about medical change are fought behind the scenes, out of hearing of the patients; but the management of troubles of the breast in this country at present lags too far behind the helpful knowledge we can now apply. The evidence regarding new treatments for breast cancer has been present for several years but ignored by too many physicians. Efforts by some doctors to bring about change have been opposed, often acrimoniously, by others.

An informed public can help expedite the new opportunities for care. If women know what questions to ask, physicians will have to pay attention, to be alert to these advances. The field of medicine is too vast, too complicated for one doctor to know all. No longer should a doctor put himself or herself in the position of understanding everything, as he or she does in answering a question with the reply: "I am the doctor. I know. Do as I say."

Women need to know, and it is my duty as a physician to speak out.

Informing the public means leveling with the public, telling the bad news as well as the good. I have already referred to the low cure rate, the high ultimate mortality among patients who have had radical mastectomies. The cure rate is so much lower than anticipated that medicine has hidden the poor result from itself. The so-called five-year cure rate as a measure of success is a shallow myth, impeding needed care that now can and should be given.

When a doctor says he has an 80 percent cure rate at five years, he neglects two things. First, that 20 percent of his patients have already died. Certainly some of these could have been saved by new methods. Second, that by ten years another 20 percent of his patients will die. Many of these too could now be saved. The new knowledge of the early widespread dissemination of the cancer cells calls for a major shift in the emphasis in treatment. (I will discuss later, in detail, the five-year cure rate and the needed shift in emphasis.)

Since the beginning of World War II, effective alternatives have appeared, used abroad more than in this country. In Finland, France, England, and Canada, radiation therapy has been found the equal to surgery in eradicating the disease in the breast and adjacent lymph nodes. There are drugs that give promise of being ultimately as effective against cancer cells as antibiotic drugs are against various bacteria.

There is already evidence that the immune defenses of the

body may some day be as useful in controlling cancer as they are in the relief and prevention of infectious diseases. Each of these will be discussed: the limited use of surgery, the newer approach of irradiation, the palliative hormones, the drugs presently available, and the prospects of immunotherapy. The nature of cancers will be described, but benign breast lumps are equally important — how they come to be and what to do about them.

The following stories of four women with breast cancer illustrate many of the problems. They show why lumps of the breast are so frightening, why even a suspicion of a lump is so upsetting, and how devastating the threat of the loss of a breast may be.

Chapter 2

Four Women

THE DISTORTIONS of life, the tragedies that carcinoma of the breast brings with it, are no secret to its victims, their families, and their friends. It attacks the center of the family, the mother, and it is the cancer most likely to strike her.

It is not only hard for the patient and her family; it is hard for the physician, too. So often he finds he is failing, and strong is the temptation to turn his back on the bad news.

(The physician I am thinking of here, and shall be writing about all through this book, can be man or woman. Fortunately, the number of women doctors is on the increase in the United States. I say "fortunately" because women should be more sensitive than men to those especial attentions women need in their medical care.)

The patient bears the brunt of the disease. The problems she faces may sometimes seem simple, but they are never easy. This was brought home to me in 1943, when three women consulted me within a six-week period for a lump in the breast. At that time I felt confident that I knew what was best to do for my patients. I was proud of the surgical skill I had to offer. I had been taught by two of the outstanding surgeons at the Massachusetts General Hospital, Dr. Edward P. Richardson and Dr. Edward D. Churchill, in the technique of a careful, thorough removal of a cancerous breast, the muscles beneath it, the lymph nodes to which it might have spread in the armpit. This operation, the radical mastectomy, was done as one piece and, insofar as possible, without ever cutting into a cancerous area. The surgery took in such a wide area that it was sometimes necessary to graft skin taken from the thigh or elsewhere to cover the chest wall.

All three women appeared to have the identical disease; all three received the identical traditional treatment. Yet the course of events for each was so different that it was obvious that their cancers must have been of different types, each needing special consideration. In spite of our knowing that such differences exist, even today one treatment — the traditional treatment by a surgical mastectomy in one form or another — continues to be the rule, recommended by the American Cancer Society and the Breast Cancer Task Force of the National Cancer Institute. What nonsense[1,2]

The first of the three patients was a tall magnificent woman of 54. Of Swedish descent, she had distinguished herself as a nurse during World War I. After the war she married and, when she was 39, had one child, a daughter. At operation, it was discerned that the lump in the patient's breast was cancerous, and that the cancer cells had spread to several of the lymph nodes in the axilla (the armpit). From outward appearances she sailed through the operation. The wound healed promptly, and she returned home after twelve days in the hospital.

I had warned her, of course, that if the lump proved at operation to be malignant, it would be only wise to carry out the radical operation, and she had agreed. But during her convalescence she started telling me of her anguish over the loss of her breast. I didn't know then why I had not heard this from other patients, but as far as I was aware, she was the first to describe to me the meaning of her breast to her as a woman. By great good luck, I sat down beside her and listened.

The second woman was ten years younger than the first. She had an excellent job as the executive secretary of a business concern in Boston, and was the main support of her aging mother. Her lump, too, proved to be malignant, and the nodes in the axilla were also involved. Her course in the hospital after operation seemed smooth and uneventful. The wound healed well and she left the hospital within two weeks, to return home to care for her mother.

She was shy, and did not unburden herself regarding the loss of her breast while she was still in the hospital. Later, as I saw her during the course of the next several years, she slowly revealed how disrupting, how depressing, it had been to have to accept the disfigurement. She had had several opportunities to get married. It was not a sexual loss that concerned her so much as a loss of a sense of being.

The third patient was a physician, aged thirty-six. She knew the sinister meaning of the easily felt large lymph nodes in her armpit: the lump in her breast presumably was a cancer and had spread not only to the lymph nodes but more widely to distant parts of the body.

At operation, the rules of surgical tradition were scrupulously followed. A piece of the lump in the breast was first excised; the pathologist reported on frozen section that the tumor was carcinoma. The biopsy wound was carefully closed. The instruments that had been used were withdrawn. The wound and skin area were soaked with tincture of iodine to kill any cell that might have been carried by the scalpel to the skin surface, and the drapes were changed. The radical operation was then carried out with freshly sterilized instruments.

I recall feeling the large nodes buried deep in the fat of the axilla beneath the pectoral muscles, and scrupulously avoiding them. Every last one was meticulously excised without any one of them being exposed, for fear that the cancerous cells might be spread. Immediately after operation one of the lymph nodes was examined by the pathologist; it appeared to be enlarged by cancer.

As we surgeons say, she withstood the operation well. That is, she promptly recovered consciousness from the anesthetic and was up and about, her arm in a firm sling. For four weeks she suffered more than the customary pain down her arm, which I attributed to my exposing the nerves leading from neck to arm when I had resected (removed surgically) the uppermost lymph nodes that the cancer might have spread to. The pain gradually subsided, as anticipated.

Six weeks after the operation the patient developed thrombosis of the brachial vein, the major vein leading upward from the arm through the armpit, to the base of the neck, and thence to the heart. The thrombosis was felt as a hard cord along the course of the vein, tender to the touch. There was some swelling of the arm, but as long as she kept her arm quiet, the swelling was not obtrusive. By the second summer after the operation, the swelling was much improved.

That summer she pricked one of her fingers while cutting roses and developed erysipelas, an acute streptococcal infection. Although the infection subsided promptly under penicillin, the inflammation accompanying the infection caused a generalized swelling of the arm, which continued from that time on, her arm swelling whenever she used it even moderately; for example, when out hiking or camping.

The early pain, the thrombosis of the arm vein, and the disastrous effect of a streptococcal infection of the hand are recognized as unfortunate complications of the radical mastectomy. The swelling of the arm persists to plague the patient to this day.

The progress of the three patients showed how little I really knew about cancer of the breast. The clinical appraisal before each operation had been the same for all three: small, presumably early cancer, and large lymph nodes, presumably enlarged by cancer. The frozen section report during operation was the same for each, and after operation the pathologist described all three tumors as being basically of the same type — invasive cancer, Grade II, arising from the cells lining the milk ducts. The cells had spread in the lymphatic vessels to the nodes of the first two patients, but had not done so in the third. The palpable, enlarged nodes in the young physician, seen under the microscope, appeared to be inflammatory, not cancerous. The decision to remove the axillary nodes along with the breast and breast muscles in the first two patients had been justifiable, but not in the third patient, the young physician. Had I broken with surgical tradition and asked the pathologist to look at some of the lymph nodes before I resected the whole mass of them, the patient would have been spared the devastating complications of the swollen and crippled arm. There were risks both ways, but my missing the chance to have done better has remained on my conscience.

Despite the similarity of the tumors described by the pathologist, the course of each of the three patients was dissimilar. The first patient gave every evidence of doing well until, one evening three years after her operation, when, as she placed a heavy pan in the oven, her arm broke at the shoulder. X-rays showed that cancer cells had spread to the bone of the upper arm and to other bones as well. This was the time when hormone treatment offered some hope, but despite its use she died four years after her operation, with extensive metastases in bones, lungs, and liver.[3] The site of the operation remained clear of any evidence of cancer. It was obvious, therefore, that cancer cells must have spread to distant parts of her body by the time the operation was performed. The discovery of the lump, and the operation, came too late to relieve her of the disease.

This hindsight can do nothing for this patient, but it can teach us much that is of use for women of the present generation, and our Swedish nurse would have cherished the thought that she was contributing now to the cause of others.

In the light of what we now know, we could have done far better; perhaps have rid her of the cancer. Certainly her life could have been prolonged, free of trouble, for several years. We have learned three things: today, faced with a patient with the same type of cancer, we know that a radical mastectomy will not cure her; that the cancer cells that have disseminated widely should be treated immediately and energetically by drugs; and, third, that instead of the mutilating mastectomy which had so upset the nurse, limited surgical removal of the tumor alone, followed by irradiation of the residual breast, will serve the breast region equally well.[4]

The second patient fared well for nine years. I saw her at stated intervals and felt encouraged by the excellent progress she was making. I tried to buoy her spirits by letting her sense my encouragement. At the beginning of the tenth year she, like the first patient, felt pain in her bones, and the cancer's spread became obvious. As further treatment, her ovaries were sterilized by x-ray and she was given male hormone, but both measures were without benefit. By this time (1954) we knew that removing the adrenal glands was helpful to some patients in this situation and, accordingly, in the eleventh year after mastectomy, I surgically removed both of her adrenal glands. This is an extensive operation, hard for the patient to bear, but she bore it stoically. Unfortunately, her cancer made little or no response; the operation only prolonged a painful, crippled existence.[5]

After the adrenalectomy she was unable to continue her job. Her one desire was to outlive her mother. Because she had become increasingly crippled, she sold the family house and moved with her mother to an apartment. There, she told me, the two of them could manage, though it would have been too much for either alone. When with me, she never complained about herself, and was always talking generously about plans for her mother. To my surprise, from her friends I learned how irritable she had become, and small wonder. Twelve years after the mastectomy she died from widespread cancer.

As with the first patient, the Swedish nurse, the antitumor drugs available today, given immediately and energetically, might well have saved her life. The cancer cells from which she died had undoubtedly passed, before the mastectomy, via the bloodstream to bones and liver, where they grew more slowly than in the first patient. They were beyond the reach of the mastectomy. She, too, need not have lost her breast. A local excision of the tumor, sparing the main part of her breast, followed by irradiation to breast and cancerous nodes, would have accomplished as much, and without the mutilation. She would have lived on, less depressed and more comfortable.

The course of events for the third patient, the young physician, differed from the other two. She never complained about her swollen crippled arm, but I knew it bothered her a great deal. She never raised an accusatory finger at me for having done more at operation than I needed to do, even though I knew she understood that her trouble resulted from excessive surgical zeal.

More difficult to handle was her desire to have another child. Six months after her operation she asked whether it was now reasonable for her to conceive again. She already had two children. We had then, as we have now, the impression that a pregnancy may stimulate the growth of any existing cancer cells. I knew she was aware of this and I didn't understand her wish for another child under such circumstances. I thought of it as a childish whim, and each time she spoke of it I put her off, suggesting, among other things, that she wait until the wound had had a longer time to heal. Finally, by the end of the second year, she insisted, and she told me why. "I feel abnormal, having lost my breast; there is something wrong. If I could have another child, it would convince me that my body is still of some use."

She started on her third pregnancy. Luckily, the pregnancy did no harm, and she lives on with her heavy arm and without her breast, otherwise well, thirty-four years following the operation. She has a right to conclude that she was cured by operation, but at the very considerable expense to her arm and her feelings about herself.

Looking back at my care of this patient, I note three things that I should do differently today. First, I would excise the segment of her breast containing the tumor, not the whole breast. After the excision I would allow the pathologist time to study the tumor, a full three days. Second, having received his report that some tumor cells were spreading out from the tumor into the adjacent breast, I would treat the remainder of the breast by high energy radiation.[4] (Radiation treatment, as we shall see, is no longer experimental but is well-founded therapy.)

When excising the tumor, I would also remove some of the lymph nodes and give them to the pathologist to check for cancer cells. I would never now excise the pectoral muscles and all of the axillary contents. That can be too disabling to the arm. If the nodes prove to contain cancer, then the axilla and other nodal areas would also be irradiated. In her case the nodes were free of disease, and she could have been spared the lifelong disability of the swollen arm.

I do not blame myself for having removed her breast at that time, for modern radiational methods had not yet been developed. To excise the tumor without removing the whole breast, to biopsy the lymph nodes without removing them all, encased in their pad of fat, would have violated an age-old surgical principle. I neither saw the need nor had the courage at that time to break with surgical tradition. But much has come to light since 1943, and to do those things today should be malpractice. Were I to care for her now she would live on well with a slightly smaller breast and a normal arm. How much easier her life!

One more of my experiences must be told to round out the complex picture.

A fourth patient had had a radical mastectomy in 1963, two years before consulting me. The surgeon, an experienced senior surgeon of an East Coast medical school, reported that the cancer had been a small one, 1 centimeter in diameter, hardly as large as a small marble, and that none of the axillary lymph nodes removed with the breast had contained cancerous cells. Both the surgeon and the pathologist told the patient and her husband that she was in the clear, with an excellent outlook, and that she was very fortunate, the cancer having been caught early, before it had spread. Now, two years after the operation, she was feeling poorly, with pain in her flank. Her doctor had found her liver enlarged, and biopsy revealed it to be full of breast cancer cells. X-ray of the spine showed a bony defect also consistent with a spread of cells from the cancer.

Both she and her husband were outraged. How could both surgeon and pathologist have been so ignorant? When the couple came to consult me they were bent on suing them both. Examination confirmed that her liver was greatly enlarged and tender, and motion of the spine painful. The mastectomy wound had healed well and there was no evidence of residual cancer in the chest wall and arm areas. As with the first two patients, the cancer cells must have fled beyond the breast to liver and bones before the operation. The mastectomy had come too late.

I took the slides of the original tumor to our pathologist, Dr. Robert Scully, and asked how it could be that a growth apparently so early and so well confined could have spread to the patient's liver and bones in such a short time. After study he pointed out that the cancer cells had penetrated into the small veins of the tumor and, presumably, had thus passed into the bloodstream without going through the lymphatic channels, a kind of spread that we now call blood vessel invasion (BVI). This, of course, was a logical explanation of what had happened, and represented a type of invasion I had encountered many years earlier with tumors of the thyroid gland. Even though the tumor was small, the radical mastectomy had indeed come too late.

She was 43 years old and her periods were continuing regularly. Castration by removal of her ovaries was advised and carried out.[3] The immediate response was dramatic. Within three weeks her liver was smaller and less tender. Over the next eight months she continued to improve, but then there came the reversal. The tumor was growing again. Bilateral adrenalectomy was performed and again she improved.[5] Before the year was out, however, the tumor was expanding once more, and rapidly. She was overwhelmed with tumor and died four years after the initial radical operation.

She was a courageous person, wonderful to take care of. She knew that she had a fatal disease and managed in an exceptional way to prepare herself for death, to deal with her fears of dying. She worried about her 18-year-old son, who, faced by the Vietnam War (it was 1967), was exposed to drugs and protest; she feared her husband was not up to helping him. He needed her. She discussed her problems freely with me, so openly and unselfishly that I was surprised to find out that at home and with her friends she, like the patient discussed above, had become increasingly critical, irritable, and demanding. It was as if she had to give way somewhere, somehow.

If we were treating her today, what would we do that is different? Several things. First, a localized excision of the tumor, removing but a small part of the breast. Second, not a frozen section diagnosis but a three-day pause for the pathologist to study the tissue adequately and, in her case, identify the invasion of the blood vessels. During this phase the patient is fully informed, given the opportunity to learn what is going on in her doctors' minds and to choose between the alternatives of treatment, surgical mastectomy or the less mutilating radiation. Third, because of the blood vessel invasion, she would be advised to accept the radiation. Fourth, since such vessel invasion indicates that cancer cells have already spread widely through the body, she would be treated immediately and energetically by drugs (which were not available at that time). Last, we can hope that she would receive more support in dealing with her emotional problems.

I must explain something about blood vessel invasion in the tumor. It cannot be identified or excluded by the pathologist during the operation by so-called frozen section. The freezing of tissue and the subsequent slicing of the icy tissue inevitably distort the patterns of the cells, and the fine points such as blood vessel invasion are rarely discernible. It takes two to three days of special staining and study to be sure of this finding, but where it exists there is no point in subjecting the patient to a radical operation or, indeed, any form of mastectomy. The alternative treatment, radiation, can eliminate cancer cells from the breast just as well as removal of the breast. What the patient needs above all else is elimination of the widely spreading tumor cells. Drugs that can effect this elimination are now available.

In summary, all four of these women were treated by radical mastectomy, the standard treatment still recommended by the American Cancer Society as the one tried and proven treatment. Three of the four patients ultimately died of the cancer despite the mastectomy. The one who survived could have been equally well treated by a simpler, less mutilating operation. Three dying, one surviving happens to be the national average for the outcome of radical mastectomy.

The patients were not chosen, however, to fit the national average. I could have selected four patients all of whom died, or four patients all of whom have survived, cured. But I chose these four because their cancers illustrate the variability of the disease and some of the problems that, if identified under modern circumstances of therapy, can be treated in a manner that results in better care and a much greater hope of cure. At the time each of the four women was operated upon, it was felt by their doctors that all had the same type of disease, that all had an equal chance of being cured. Now we know better and can do better.

After we have discussed the everyday troubles that women have with their breasts — thickenings, cysts, and benign lumps, their relation to the ovarian cycle, their identification and control — we shall return to cancer, to the important new knowledge and reasons for the new hope in treatment, the meaning of the critical pathology in such matters as invasion of blood vessels, where surgery may be replaced by irradiation, the new drugs, and thoughts about how the life of the patient may be made more tolerable and comfortable.

Chapter 3

The Biology of
the Normal Breast
and Its Everyday Troubles

As WE START, we must be sure of our terms. Words used in everyday speech must be dissociated from medical terms with quite specific meanings. "Tumor," for example, to many means "cancer," but in medicine it doesn't mean this at all. Medically, a "tumor" is a swelling: perhaps a bruise with a pooling of blood beneath it, a localized infection, an abscess, a cyst, or a growth of cells. A tumor, therefore, may or may not be threatening. Because the term has been used at times instead of the frightening word "cancer," some people think it always has a sinister connotation, and this is quite misleading and undeserved.

"Benign" and "malignant" also need careful definition. Benign means "harmless." A benign tumor is one that, if allowed to go untreated, will not endanger life. Malignant, to the contrary, means "harmful." A malignant tumor, if not attended to, will sooner or later do damage, and ultimately it will kill the person harboring it.

Medicine has its own specific terms, which have a way of straying into casual conversation and press releases, often in a misleading way. I have in mind such words as "neoplasia" and "hyperplasia," "adenoma," "papilloma," "fibroma" and "lipoma," "carcinoma" and "sarcoma." Each has its definite meaning and its place in describing the troubles of the breast, as we shall see.

The breast is an astonishingly complicated organ, an inseparable part of the whole intricate system of reproduction. It grows throughout pregnancy, ready to do its job the minute the child is born. When no longer needed to supply the infant's nutrition, it recedes, to start all over again when called on by another pregnancy. Man has nothing like it.

Imagine thousands, tens of thousands, of tiny cells able to secrete milk on order.[1] Each cell must absorb, from the blood flowing by, all the basic substances it needs to make colostrum and milk. The basic substances are water, salts, sugar, fats, and small nitrogen-containing molecules. These are put together inside the cell to make the complicated, life-building fluids. Colostrum, the glistening, clear fluid that is the first to be secreted at childbirth, contains immunity-providing proteins that protect against measles and mumps and other infections until the infant can build his or her own immunities. Milk, appearing a day later, contains in addition a balanced amount of calcium, magnesium, and phosphorus to build the bones of the infant, protein and sugar for the tissues to grow and live on. There is a full score of vitamins, and cream in the right amount for the human infant.

The milk-secreting gland cells are not the only complicated part of the breast. There are the ducts that carry the milk from glands to nipple — the pipeline system. The milk secreted by the glands passes out of the cells into a tiny collecting chamber, an alveolus. Thence the milk is carried by a system of ducts, arranged like the branches of a tree, to the ampulla, the collecting vestibule immediately beneath the nipple. From the ampulla the infant gets a generous, sometimes overgenerous, mouthful at the start of suckling.

The ducts and their lining cells have specific, well-defined duties. They must grow lengthwise as the breast develops during pregnancy. They must convey the milk promptly when called on. The cry of the hungry infant from rooms away may start the flow of the milk, or the flow may await stimulation of the nerves from nipple to brain by the suckling of the infant. All this is subject to the direction of the mother's nervous system.

There are many complicated links between the breast and the

rest of the body. Crampy contractions of the uterus are induced by nursing in the first days after birth of the child. These cramps, also mediated through the brain, help complete the shrinking down of the uterus. And when feedings become less frequent, somehow the breast knows how to adapt, providing less and less milk.

As the breast recedes after lactation, not only the old gland cells, but the unneeded cells of the ducts must somehow be dissolved and gotten rid of, making a place for the new cells that will come with the next pregnancy. A clean-up job like this may not seem as difficult as the making of the milk, yet it is interesting to note at this point that the ducts appear to get into more trouble than the gland cells. Three fourths of all the malignant tumors of the breast are believed to originate in the duct cells, only one-fourth in the gland cells.

In addition to ducts and gland cells, there is fibrous tissue that supports and contains the breast. This tissue gives rise to more doubts and fears than the glands and ducts together, for it is the most common source of lumps in the breast. It is, however, rarely the site of malignant tumors.

The fibrous tissue attaches the breast to the chest wall and, like a basket, keeps the breast from sagging downward unduly. Other fibers hold the segments of the breast together and support the ducts. All of the fibers elongate and increase in number as the breast grows in pregnancy; they expand further with lactation. At the end of milking, they know somehow to retract and return to their former size.

The fibrous tissue of the breast is a first cousin of the muscle of the uterine wall. In pregnancy the uterine wall grows enormously to house the infant and to play its part in expelling the baby when the pregnancy is completed. Afterward, it atrophies to almost its previous size. Both uterus and breast respond to the same ovarian hormones. The breast also has a special stimulating hormone from the pituitary, prolactin, which aids the growth of the breast during pregnancy and the making of milk. The two organs grow simultaneously during pregnancy. When pregnancy is past, the uterus dwindles first; the breast awaits the end of lactation. The waxing and waning of both the uterine muscle and the fibrous tissue of the breast throughout the menstrual cycle run parallel in the two organs.

The troubles of the uterine muscle and the fibrous tissue of the breast are also much akin; fibroids of the uterus are first cousins of the fibrous lumps of the breast. They grow at the same times and both disappear after the menopause. Malignant growths in the fibrous tissue of either are rare.

The fourth tissue of the breast is fat. Fat cells cushion the organ, and make it comfortable as well as graceful. The fat cells are found within the capsule of the breast itself, between the lobules of the glands, in between ducts, and in the ampulla under the nipple. They are also found outside the capsule of the breast between breast and skin, as fat is found under the skin over almost the entire body. Occasionally, conglomerations of fat cells form, and, if encapsulated, are called a "lipoma"; but seldom are fat cells a source of malignancy. Fat is the most harmless of the breast tissues.

Lymphoid cells are found here and there in the breast as they are, indeed, found in most glands of the body. These cells are a part of our immunologic system. They may help in the scavenging of outworn cells, but, more important, they arrest infection that may come from bacteria swimming up the ducts from the nipple or arriving by the bloodstream. In some conditions they are found in excessive numbers; it is believed that this increase represents an effort by the body to stem some abnormal condition, such as the start of a cancer. They are for the most part considered welcome guardians of our health. Rarely, if ever, do they create a lump in the breast on their own.

Outside the breast, lymph cells are found in nearly every tissue, predominantly in lymph nodes, thymus, and spleen. The lymph nodes relating to the breast are found in the axilla, in the hollow above the collarbone (the supraclavicular fossa), along the blood vessels beneath the breastbone (the internal mammary vessels), and at the neck of the ribs (in the chest wall at the back). The lymph fluid of the breast flows to all these four areas.

Lymph nodes have multiple functions. They act as sieves. The lymphatic fluid flowing to and through them is filtered of bacteria, cast-off cells, and any other particulate matter. Cancer cells are caught as they drift up the lymphatic vessels. The nodes also nurture such cancerous cells, many of which take root within them. From these colonies in the nodes, cancer cells may later be carried by the bloodstream to distant organs of the body — lungs, liver, bones, and brain.

The lymphatic tissue is also believed to build immunity proteins and, like the lymph cells within the breast itself, to maintain our resistance to infections.

The body has a miraculous control over the amount of blood flowing into a tissue, and the return flows of blood and lymph. The rate of circulation is maintained at a level sufficient to meet the metabolic needs of each tissue. When the metabolism of the breast is elevated by hormonal stimulation, the blood flow increases. This can be appreciated by the woman as a fullness, warmth, and sometimes a tenderness. The rise in metabolic rate and the increase of blood flow in the breast are greatest in pregnancy, and the woman who has already experienced one pregnancy knows that if these feelings continue past the time of her expected period, the breast itself indicates a probable pregnancy. Soon a colostrum-like fluid will be expressible from the nipple.

A rise in metabolic rate and increase in blood flow occur with each menstrual cycle. The stimulation during the first half of the cycle is by the female hormone of the ovary, estrogen. This hormone stimulates the production of new cells, gland cells, duct cells, and fibrous tissue cells. Immediately after ovulation the second ovarian hormone, progesterone, is added. Progesterone initiates the secreting process in the gland cells. Even this limited stimulation of the breast can be felt by many women. Part of the swelling is the actual blood increase, and part of it is the greater amount of fluid seeping out of the capillaries into the tissues. When pregnancy does not take place and the hormonal process is reversed, the arterial flow diminishes abruptly. The venous and lymphatic returns overtake the production of fluid; the amount decreases. And the breasts soften.

These changes in blood flow and consequent changes in warmth explain why thermography, the recording of temperatures, can be used to register the metabolic rate of the breast or of parts of the breast.[2] If there is an abscess or a rapidly growing tumor, the blood flow to that part is increased, and appears on the thermogram as a hot spot.

The breast also contains sensory nerves, which bear a special relation to control of breast function. We have already referred to the cry of the infant and the effect of suckling on the production and flow of milk and on the contractions of the uterus after birth. The nerve stimulus from the nipple passes to the special spot of the forebrain, the supraoptic nucleus, where the oxytoxic hormone is secreted.[3] This hormone released into the bloodstream in turn stimulates the flow of the milk and the contractions of the uterine muscles. The stimulus to the brain also releases the hormones that produce milk, prolactin especially.[4,5]

Perhaps the most intricate and least understood system of the breast is its hormonal development and control. The growth, maturation, and function of the breast are the result of a sequential stimulation by several separate hormones. Four glands secrete these hormones: the ovary, anterior pituitary, adrenal cortex, and thyroid, all governed by the brain as part of bodily development and adult function. The development of the breast starts at puberty, continues during adolescence, and reaches adult size as body growth is completed.

Young girls have few troubles with their breasts during the years of development. When they reach maturity and the menstrual cycle starts, troubles may begin. The growth stimulus may go beyond adjustment and lumps may appear. Seldom cancerous in the woman in her 20s or 30s, the lumps can be a source of anxiety and need to be understood.

Reversible Troubles – The Fibrocystic Changes

If acute infections and caking of the breast during lactation are excluded, the most common trouble affecting women's breasts is by all odds the fibrocystic disorder.[6,7,8] Fully half of women in the United States have it at some time or other in their lives. For some, the disorder is troublesome enough to warrant attention, but for most, the trouble is reversible and undergoes a spontaneous remission, so it frequently passes unnoticed.

The disorder is an exaggeration of the changes that normally take place in the breasts with each menstrual cycle, but only during the active phase of menstrual ovarian life. It is to a large extent self-limited, and is relieved by a pregnancy, the arrival of the menopause, or even by the lessening of tension in a hectic life. Since the disorder appears in large part to be generated by long successions of menstrual cycles uninterrupted by pregnancies, the social policy of birth control accounts for some of its prevalence today, and its incidence is likely to increase further in the foreseeable future. It appears in the breasts in a variety of forms, depending on which of the tissues react most to the stimulation: the fibrous tissue, the glands, or the ducts. Because of this variability, it goes by several different names, including, among others, the older terms "chronic cystic mastitis" or "mastasia," and the new terms "sclerosing adenosis" and "ductal dysplasia." Finally, because of its frequent confusion with the much less common and far more serious cancerous growths, it is important that we examine the disorder in detail so that women can learn how to differentiate the two — the common and innocuous from the less common and harmful.

Young women are often startled by the presence of the common lumpiness and they should realize its origins and character. Carcinoma is rare in women under 35, and women should not be unduly frightened by lumpiness that is encountered in their early years.

When a woman is in her 40s, the age when cancers may begin to appear, it is particularly important that both she and her physician understand the nature of the fibrocystic disorder. For example, in the last years of her ovarian life she may develop cysts, which will plague her by raising the specter of a cancer.

Typically, both breasts are to some extent involved. They feel fuller, heavier, and a bit lumpy, and are also warm and tender in spots. Women who notice such changes during their normal menstrual cycle are especially likely to be aware of any exaggeration of these changes if they develop the disorder. The lumpiness and tenderness are found most often in the outer aspect of the breast, particularly in the upper portion near the armpit, simply because there is more breast tissue in this part of the breast.

The normal preparation for pregnancy and lactation overshoots, causing thickening and lumpiness. What starts out as an orderly process is carried too far to be resorbed when the pregnancy does not take place, so each month an excess is built up. The breast, unlike the uterus, is unable to shed promptly its preparation for pregnancy. It has to resorb the cells, whereas the uterus casts off the cells in menstruation.

Although thickening of both breasts is usual, single sections, or lobules, may often be felt, each section leading by a single duct to the nipple. The overgrowth may involve only fibrous tissue, or it may involve the cells of ducts and glands as well. If there is a lot of gland proliferation, it can be recognized on the modern Xeromammograms, or by microscopic examination of a small sample (a biopsy) by the pathologist. He may call it sclerosing adenosis, or fibroadenomatosis. When the chief problem lies in the ducts, it is called ductal dysplasia. The ductal proliferation can sometimes be felt, particularly in the ampulla beneath the areola of the nipple, and a Xeromammogram shows the thickening of the ducts in this area.

Lumpiness may be produced not only by proliferation of cells, but also by the collection of fluids, which leads to formation of cysts. Usually the cysts are small and multiple, but occasionally may be the size of a golf ball or larger. Basically the fluid is colostrum, together with the undissolved debris of discarded cells. The cysts, because of their local character, arouse the greatest suspicion of a cancer although in themselves they are usually harmless. If fluid can be withdrawn from the lump with a needle and syringe, we know it is a cyst and not a solid tumor.

When considering the diagnosis, the doctor should examine the uterus as well as the breast, and should take a vaginal smear. When the smear is studied, special attention should be given to the character of the cells and to the degree of hormonal stimulation. Since the hormonal process that induces the fibrocystic disorder also affects the uterus, comparable change is generally to be found simultaneously in both organs, uterus as well as breast. Thus, women in whom fibrocystic changes persist over several months are often found to have fibroids of the uterus. Indeed, one of the ways to substantiate the diagnosis of fibrocystic disorder in the breast is to determine whether the uterus is enlarged generally or harbors one or more fibroid tumors. Forty percent of women in their 40s have such uterine changes. Obviously, such problems are most likely to occur in women at times of maximum ovarian activity, particularly in the early years, 18 to 25, the period of greatest fertility. They are less prominent in the years when women are having their children, but reappear during the 40s, when irregularities begin to occur in the hormone balance.

There are seasonal variations in fibrocystic problems much as there are in the breast changes during the normal menstrual cycle. From December to May the activity of the breast in most women is most noticeable. This is the season when, apparently, the ovaries are at peak activity. It is the season of greatest fertility of women in the northern hemisphere. Those normal women who notice swelling and tenderness of their breasts in the week before the onset of menstruation are likely to notice the fibrocystic lumpiness most often in these same months.

In our complicated society, there are many other influences that may interfere with the normal ovarian cycle. Sexual interest and anticipation can be another stimulator of ovarian activity. Anxieties and disappointments can induce the reverse.

Fibrocystic changes may also be exaggerated if the menstrual cycle becomes irregular, particularly if there is a prolonged interval in the cycle. If ovulation fails to occur, fluid may accumulate and cysts form or refill. This is most often encountered in the second half of the summer, and accounts for those women who find their greatest lumpiness in late August and September. It is a problem encountered by many women as they approach the menopause. The lumpiness slowly disappears after the menopause, but may be reactivated by the use of estrogens. These seasonal changes are not absolute, but awareness of them helps patient and physician to understand what is happening.

Women can help themselves and their physicians if they will pay attention to the changes that occur in their breasts with each menstrual cycle. The program of the American Cancer Society urging women to learn self-examination is a sound concept, but it is essential that women who carry out self-examination understand the history of the normal breast and the possible development of fibrocystic disease. In this way they will not become unduly alarmed by normal changes, yet will recognize "something different," which their doctor should check.

As women reach maturity, they will do well to check their breasts themselves on some kind of a regular basis. (How to carry out the breast self-examination is described on page 205.) The check is best made as the menstrual period is ending, for two reasons. First, menstruation will have reminded the woman and, second, it is the phase when the breasts are least swollen. Should a cyst or a solid tumor have developed, it is most easily identified in this phase of the cycle.

If a young woman finds a lump she may wait to see what happens following her next period, since in a young woman cancer is highly unlikely. If the lump is a cyst, it may resolve after a cycle or two and disappear. If, however, the lump persists, she should go to her doctor.

A woman past 30 who has not previously had a cyst should report to her doctor when the lump is first felt. This is to make certain that the lump is benign, not a carcinoma.

It is difficult for the woman and, indeed, difficult for the doctor to identify the nature of all lumps. Hardness and tenderness are by no means certain signs of any specific type of lump. The only sign that the woman can depend on is that fibrocystic lumps wax and wane with the menstrual cycle. Cancerous lumps do not.

There is also security in numbers. If the breast is diffusely lumpy, all lumps being approximately equal, the lumps are not cancerous. A woman should be alert to a single lump no matter how small.

Obviously it is of paramount importance for the woman who has a lump or lumps in her breast to be sure that the right diagnosis is arrived at and that the doctor takes every available means to come to the diagnosis before resorting to surgical biopsies. Careful attention to the history and to the physical character of the lumps can carry the doctor a long way to the correct diagnosis. In addition, he has now greater refinements of visualizing the breast by x-ray and other means. It is no longer as necessary as it was ten years ago to resort to surgical diagnostic biopsies.

This matter of making the correct diagnosis will be considered further in Chapter 12. But first we must consider the tumors, the neoplasms, both benign and malignant.

Chapter 4

Breast Tumors, Benign and Malignant

THE WORRISOME TUMORS of the breast are the localized, unrestrained growths of new cells. The multiplication of the cells starts in one spot of one or the other breast, almost never in two spots or a spot in both breasts at the same time. In contrast, the cell proliferations described in the previous chapter, which were exaggerations of normal expected processes, were always diffuse, involving to some degree all of the particular tissue throughout both breasts. Medicine calls the localized new cell growths "neoplasms," from the Greek meaning "new tissue"; the diffuse cell proliferations discussed in Chapter 3 are called "hyperplasias," also from the Greek: "a greater number of cells." The hyperplasias characteristically wax and wane under hormone control. The neoplasms are basically an unrestrained growth of cells, only a few of which are influenced by hormones.

The new growths, or neoplasms, may be benign or malignant. The benign growths are constrained by a capsule and give trouble only by the pressure they induce and the worry they engender about their nature. The malignant cells know no bounds, and invade the tissues of the breast and far parts of the body, disrupting the functions of organs as they grow.

Benign Neoplasms

Small, solid, isolated, single, benign lumps are sometimes encountered in the breasts of women during their active ovarian years. They are true neoplasms because they are formed by continuing multiplication of new cells in one spot. They are benign because the cells are confined by a fibrous capsule and do not wander into or invade the breast.[1] When made of fibrous cells alone, they are called "fibromas"; when they consist of gland cells, they are "adenomas"; if of mixed cells, "fibroadenomas." Such neoplasms have a smooth fibrous capsule, no tentacles, and are therefore loosely attached and surprisingly movable within the breast. They contrast with the fibrocystic lumps mentioned in Chapter 3, which are true segments of the breast and are firmly attached. Such segments are more like pieces of a pie, more triangular than round, flat in front and behind, where they lie against the chest wall. The neoplasm grows in all directions and tends, therefore, to be round.

The benign neoplasms are for the most part complications of fibrocystic hyperplasia and are therefore encountered most often when the fibrocystic disorder is at its height, usually in young women, aged 18 to 25. They are rarely encountered in women in their 30s and 40s and almost never after the menopause. If found after the menopause, they have probably been there from earlier years. They are usually slow-growing and for that reason are still small when found, each the size of a small grape. If they are overlooked in a large breast, they may reach a considerable size, perhaps that of a plum. As far as we know now, they do not change into malignant neoplasms. The only cure is surgical removal. Except to give the woman the comfort of knowing, of being sure what they are, there is no urgency about cutting them out.

Such fibromas are related to the rounded fibroid tumors of the uterus. Those with gland cells in them, the fibroadenomas of the breast, are akin to the uterine fibroids, which include the gland cells of the uterine lining, the so-called fibroendotheliomas. Fibroids of the uterus can be expected to atrophy after the menopause. It is possible that the same thing would happen to a breast fibroma, but it has not to my knowledge been put to the test. It has always been important to remove the lump to be sure of its nature. In contrast, the diagnosis of the uterine fibroid is easier and more secure. The physician can identify the characteristic tumor on pelvic examination, and a normal Pap smear indicates that it does not contain a cancer. It may therefore be left alone. As noted before, fibromas of the breast and uterus rarely, if ever, become malignant.

Malignant Neoplasms

The malignant neoplasms of the breast, unrestrained in their growth, are of two kinds — sarcomas and carcinomas. They form from different tissues and have quite different biologic histories.[2]

Sarcoma of the breast is a most unusual tumor. It is an unbridled growth of the fibrous tissue that characteristically occurs in adolescents and young women. Sarcoma is the name attached to all malignant tumors of fibrous tissue origin; in general such tumors occur in younger people. For example, the malignant tumors of bone called "osteogenic sarcoma" occur in children and adolescents. Sarcomas are so unusual in the breast that physicians seldom see more than a very few. Still, rare as they are, they have to be kept in mind. In general, they are rapid-growing and invasive, their cells spreading early via the bloodstream throughout the body.

Carcinoma is the term applied to malignant tumors originating in specialized tissues, such as ducts and glands. Carcinoma is the medical term for cancer, and cancer in turn derives from the Latin word meaning "crab." Typically, carcinomas spread in unrestrained fashion along paths that come to resemble the legs of crabs. They not only spread locally, but also by devious means travel in the blood and lymph streams and along nerves to other parts of the body. In contrast to sarcomas, these tumors occur during the older decades. Carcinomas of the breast are rare before the age of 30 and continue to be so in the 30s and 40s. Their incidence increases as age advances and they are therefore related in some way to the aging process.

A few general considerations regarding carcinoma of the breast: With the exception of skin cancer, it is the most common malignant neoplasm afflicting women in the United States, Canada, England, and western Europe. Official statistics vary from country to country, and, within the United States, from federal public health to state health departments and cancer societies. The lowest reported incidence of breast cancer in the lifetime of a woman is 1 in 18, or 5 percent; the highest, 1 in 14, or 7 percent.

Carcinoma of the breast is not one disease; there are at least fifteen distinct, separate varieties.[1] They vary from sluggish growths to rapidly spreading tumors. The growth of some is so sluggish, the cells so slow to invade outward, that they border on benign. Indeed, there is an interphase between the clearly benign and clearly malignant.

The most frequent tumors of the interphase are minute islands, or clusters, of cells too small to be felt or seen by the naked eye. These are sometimes called "multicentric foci," in reference to the several little spots. Under the microscope the cells of these islands are larger than normal cells and look like cancer cells; but they fail to develop into a growing, spreading tumor. They occur in perhaps as many as 30 percent of women at the age of 50. Little is understood of their real nature. I mention them not because I think them dangerous, but because there is much controversy about them. Some surgeons feel that breasts containing such islands should be removed for fear the islands may later start growing and develop into true cancers.[3]

Comparable tiny clusters of cancer-like cells appear in other organs, such as the thyroid and the prostate, where we have learned to leave them alone because we know them to be innocuous.[4]

If one of these clusters is found in the breast, there are usually more, often many more, and not in one but in both breasts. These little clusters of odd-looking cells give rise to great indecision, frustration, and difference of opinion among doctors as to their meaning and practical consequences. From a statistical point of view, they can't all be cancers or the seeds of real cancers. If they were, cancers of the breast would be much more common, afflicting 20 to 30 percent of women; yet clinical breast cancer is relatively uncommon, 7 percent or less on the average. We shall come back to this problem of multicentric foci of cancer-like cells when we are talking about treatment.

The first order of tumors that must be considered malignant is a group of cancers in which the cells slowly multiply but appear still to be restrained by an anatomic barrier, such as the outer membrane of a duct or of a glandular alveolus. The cells multiply like cancer cells, but lack the invasive power to penetrate the membrane (Ackerman Type I[1]). Sometimes they are multiple. These tumors are readily cured by a simple surgical excision. Only the local tumor needs to be excised. It is not necessary to remove the breast. In this group are such tumors as the intraductal carcinoma, the papillary carcinoma, and the lobular alveolar carcinoma. These make up about 5 to 10 percent of all breast carcinomas in the United States and western Europe.

The next group of cancers is clearly invasive, but sluggishly so. The cells have the power to penetrate the duct or alveolar membranes and to continue proliferating outside the confines of the original cell growth (Ackerman Type II[1]). If sufficient time has elapsed for these migrant cells to wander far into the breast, they may not be removed by simple excision but will need either the addition of radiation or the removal of the entire breast. The young physician, the third patient described in Chapter 2, had a cancer of this type. These tumors make up approximately 10 percent of the total breast cancers.

The next two types of breast cancers are more unrestrained; the cells are prone to embark on distant invasion (Ackerman Type III[1]). The majority arise from cells of the ducts and are called "invasive ductal carcinomas"; the minority come from the gland cells and are called "adenocarcinomas." Together they constitute about 65 percent of all breast cancers in the United States, Canada, and western Europe. The cells of these types invade more rapidly than those described above and spread throughout the breast. Many of them are also caught up in the lymphatic vessels and are to be found in the lymph nodes draining the breast. Few if any of these cancers are eradicated by local treatment of the breast and lymph nodes, either by surgery or by irradiation. By the time the primary tumor is recognized by the woman or her doctor, cells have already spread into the bloodstream by way of the lymph nodes or directly from the tumor into the blood. Sooner or later, perhaps years later, these tumors prove fatal, not from recurrence of the cancer in the breast region, but from the cells that have spread to the liver, lungs, and bones. In the first two patients of Chapter 2, the cells had escaped from the tumor to the distant organs before their sources in the breast and lymph nodes were removed by the mastectomy.

A fourth type of cancer, which accounts for some 15 percent of breast cancers, includes those cancers with cells that have a predilection for invading the small veins within the primary tumor, passing directly into the bloodstream and spreading early throughout the body (Ackerman Type IV[1]). The fourth patient whose history was recounted in Chapter 2 had a tumor of this type. Seemingly, at the time of her operation she had a good prognosis. The tumor in the breast was small and its cells appeared to be proliferating in a relatively sluggish fashion. However, the cells had early invaded the veins and spread before the tumor was felt and the breast removed. Before a year was up, the patient's liver was found to be full of cancer. By the fourth year, she was dead. The outlook for patients with these hitherto lethal breast cancers is now altogether different since the appearance of antitumor drugs. Immediate and prolonged administration of drugs, as practiced over the last five years, has already benefited many patients with early spread of cancer.

Another of the most virulent of breast cancers, fortunately rare, making up not more than 5 percent of the cases, is the so-called inflammatory cancer. It spreads rapidly, like an infectious cellulitis or carbuncle. Surgeons have long known that attempts to cut it out only spread it farther.[5] The effect of irradiation is uncertain, and drugs thus far have failed to do more than temporarily stem its growth.

Although we don't know why or how a cell becomes cancerous, we do realize that cancerous cells proliferate at different rates. The rate of growth is called the "doubling time" — the time needed for one cell to grow to two, two to four, four to eight, and so on.[6,7] Compared with other cancers, the doubling times of breast cancers are moderately slow, ranging from 50 to 150 days. Since it takes approximately twenty doubling times for a cancer to reach 1 centimeter in diameter (the size of a small marble), the fastest-growing breast cancers spend 1000 days, or nearly three years, in reaching that size. Since it is unusual for a cancer of the breast to be discovered by either the patient or examining physician when it is less than 1 centimeter in diameter, most breast cancers have existed for three years or longer by the time they are first found. This is a long period for such a tumor to be growing, and one can see the possibility that the tumor, at its twelfth or fifteenth doubling time, before it can be felt, may have given off cells into the tissue channels, cells that are then carried to far-off parts of the body.

There, in the liver or bones, doubling presumably at the same rate as in the parent tumor, the metastasis may spend years before it becomes large enough to be appreciated. If it takes three years for a tumor to grow large enough to be recognized in the breast, its daughter cells in the liver will not be appreciated at 1 centimeter, and it may take additional years before the cancer in the liver is recognized.

This long delay between the spread of the cells from the tumor in the breast to organs elsewhere in the body is the reason so many years may elapse between the removal of the cancer in the breast and the recognition of that same cancer elsewhere in the body.[8]

This is a reason that the concept of the "five-year cure" can be so misleading. The doubling time is a guide, but not an absolute. Breast cancers, indeed many cancers, may not grow at a steady rate. There may well be fluctuations, phases of rapid growth followed by phases of sluggish growth. It is also quite likely, as we know from observation of animal tumors, that cells on the surface of the tumor grow more rapidly than those in the interior. In the deep recesses of the tumor they may be shut off from a sufficient blood supply and lie dormant for long periods.

The essential characteristic of the malignant neoplasm is that its cells keep on multiplying in unrestrained fashion and don't know to stay at home. They wander forth, and if the climate and ground are propitious, a single cell or a cluster of cells may set up housekeeping, sometimes near at home but more often far away, in other tissues. If enough such new homes are settled in other organs far away and the clusters grow to sizable satellites, the function of the organ and the life of the host is snuffed out.

The path along which cancer cells most often spread out from the original tumor is the tissue spaces of the breast itself. Second is the lymphatic vessels and thus to the lymph nodes of the breast region. Next in frequency are the blood vessels and then the nerve sheaths.

The most direct route of spread to other organs is through the blood, but the spread also occurs from the lymph nodes, either by continuing in the flow of the lymph from the lymph node into the bloodstream or by invading the blood vessels within the lymph nodes.[9,10]

Once outside, in the body, breast cancer cells have a predilection for settling and growing in the bone marrow, the liver, and the lungs. Occasionally breast cancer cells also settle in the brain, the ovaries, or the adrenals, but seldom in such organs as the kidney or the thyroid (favorite sites for other cancers).

One peculiarity of the spread of breast cancer cells to the bone marrow is that the cells go only to the "warm bones," such as the pelvis, spine, ribs, and skull, rather than to the "cold bones" of the hands, lower arms, feet, and lower legs. The cold environment is not a hospitable one for the growth of the cancer cells.

The structure of the tumor and the manner in which the cancer cells appear to be spreading do not tell us everything about the cancer's virulence. There are many influences that are still obscure, among them the causes of the cancers and the counterforces raised by the patient's body. If causes, especially direct causes, were known and the causes could be eliminated, obviously women could be protected in advance. Despite much new knowledge regarding the causes of animal cancers and of some malignant tumors of the human body, surprisingly little of a substantial nature has been uncovered about human breast cancer.

Chemicals found to cause malignant tumors of other organs, such as the bladder, have not been identified in patients who have developed breast tumors.[11] In recent months environmental poisons have been widely incriminated as causes of some cancers, but no specific irritant to the breast has been found.[12]

Radiation, known to excite malignancy in other organs, has been scrutinized as a possible cause.[13] A group of young women with tuberculosis of the lung whose breasts had been exposed to an unusual amount of x-ray because of the repeated chest examinations did indeed have a greater than expected incidence of breast cancer in later years.[14] But if x-ray is an influence, it must be slight, for x-rays of the chest are common and the number of women exposed to many chest plates and fluoroscopies who have developed cancer is small.

Women often ask about trauma to the breast, either from a blow or a sore spot that might be caused by a tight bra. Blunt trauma to the breast is not infrequent, and is occasionally followed by a swollen clot. Still, there is no evidence that this leads either sooner or later to the formation of a cancer.

They ask about diet. There is a possibility that the difference in diet between the United States and Japan is a factor in the much lower incidence of breast cancer in Japanese women. But if this is so, we do not know what the specific chemical may be.[15] Still, although a chemical substance has not been identified, it would be as wrong to dismiss a good diet as unimportant as it would be to dismiss general health as unimportant. Health is important to the body's resistance to infections, intestinal ulcers, degenerative diseases, and other disorders. If immunologic resistance proves to be important in the body's battle against cancer, as many think it is, then such matters as diet, sleep, and composure should be important in forestalling cancer anywhere in the body.

A virus found in the milk of certain mice has been proven to be the means of transmission of breast cancer from the mother mouse to her offspring.[16] Despite many searches, no such virus has as yet been identified in the human being.[17]

The cancer-stimulating effects of the various hormones have been studied[18] largely because of the wide use of the Pill and of female hormones at the menopause and after. Though hormones may increase the susceptibility to cancer and perhaps initiate cancer in the uterus and vagina, evidence is lacking that they themselves directly cause cancer of the breast. The duration of the active ovarian life, the age of the initial pregnancy, and use of the Pill may also be of indirect influence. All of these will be dealt with later in detail.

Other glands, too, may well be involved. The pituitary secretes prolactin and there is some evidence that an excess may be harmful by stimulating abnormal breast growth.[19] We are as yet unsure of this. Women who have low thyroid function are believed by some physicians to be slightly more susceptible to breast cancer than the normal woman.[20] Such women are prone to continued secretion of a watery milk, a condition called "galactorrhea." Some hold that this may be a premonitory sign of breast cancer. Whether or not low thyroid function is deleterious to the breast, it is important for other reasons to maintain a normal thyroid level. This is readily done by thyroid medication. Otherwise the heart may suffer from the low function.

Of all the causes and influences, there remain the genetic. Strains of mice and rats have been identified whose offspring either frequently or seldom develop breast cancer.[16] In the human being, certain families have been found in which the women have a greater than average incidence of breast cancer.[21] The tendency appears to be genetic because it may be transmitted down the family tree through the father as well as the mother. This is scary to the women who have cancer in their families, but fortunately such inheritance is rare and the likelihood of a person's developing the familial cancer is far from certain, statistical reports and press releases to the contrary. We shall deal with this genetic factor in Chapter 5.

Although this summary of possible cancers and influences

may seem short and cursory, there is no doubt that the search for causes is of the utmost significance. Undoubtedly there is not just one cause, and not one aggravating factor. There are multiple contingencies known and suspected, and as these are unraveled, treatment will become less and less hit-or-miss and more and more secure. Measures for prevention may even become possible. Ultimately the most important forces for evil and good may turn out to lie in the cells of the breast themselves and of the patient's body as a whole.

For example, we have reason to believe that the body sets up a counterforce against many of the cancers, and the lymphatic system seems at times to be related to such counteraction.[22] This theoretical immune force may have been the reason why the course of events of each of the first two patients described in the second chapter differed from one another, why the first patient succumbed at the end of the fourth year while the second survived for twelve years. Seemingly the structure and type of spread of both tumors were the same at the time the operations were performed. The theory is that the first patient had little resistance to her tumor; the second had considerable resistance until it finally gave way in the tenth year.

The third of our patients, the one who survives free of tumor, thirty-four years after operation, may well have developed a strong resistance or counterforce to the tumor. The lymph nodes draining the area of the tumor were enlarged, not with cancer but by a lymphoid process that may well have held the tumor in abeyance.

The fourth patient, the woman whose tumor cells had invaded the small veins and spread early to the liver, presumably had an entirely different type of inner reaction. The tumor cells were attracted to the blood vessels. If there was any restraint on the part of the body, it was unable to deflect this spread from the vessels. As one looks at the four patients and the type of tumor each had, it is clear that one treatment is no longer suitable for all women with cancers of the breast.

Chapter 5

Who Gets Cancer of the Breast?

AN ASTOUNDING FACT about breast cancer in women is that the frequency of its occurrence has not changed materially in the United States over the past forty years. Despite all the recent publicity from the National Cancer Institute, the American Cancer Society, and the news media, when the number of women is taken into account, at the most only 1 of 14 women develop the cancer. One in 14 is but 7 percent, and that is essentially where it was ten, twenty, thirty, and forty years ago.[1-5]

The determination in the United States of the incidence of breast cancer in women — that is, the number of women in terms of the total woman population who have developed breast cancer — has been possible only in the last forty years. Breast cancer was not a reportable disease forty years ago, so the figures of the incidence for that time were in part an estimate. An accurate count of women afflicted with the cancer was made in 1937 in ten large urban communities distributed across the country, and from these counts an estimate was made for the entire country. Assuming that the estimates of forty and thirty years ago were accurate, and subsequent studies indicate that they were close, the occurrence of the cancer has not materially changed since 1937.[2] There is a suggestion that the cancer has appeared in more younger women since 1930; this may be due to the two-year-earlier onset of menstruation that has taken place in the generation born after 1930.[4,5]

For this forty-year period, 1937 to 1977, the incidence of breast cancer in the United States is variously quoted between 1 woman in 14 and 1 in 18. One in 14 is given by the National Cancer Institute, and 1 in 15 by the American Cancer Society.[4,5] (Strax and Johnson, in their books on health care, say 1 in 15.[6,7]) One in 15 equals 6.6 percent; 1 in 14, 7.14 percent. I have chosen the outside figures of 1 in 14, approximately 7 percent of the female population.

The American Cancer Society and the various agencies talking and writing about breast cancer are not saying that breast cancer has increased. They are calling our attention to breast cancer in an effort to get women and physicians to be aware of the possibility of its occurrence, asking women to examine themselves and to report any symptom early to the physician, when care is most likely to be successful. To this end they are successful, but at the same time they are frightening many women more than is needed to get them to pay attention. Cancer of the breast is not threatening as many women as the agencies make it sound. A young woman looking ahead to her life does not need to be frightened by the prospect. Should she by chance be one of the few who develop the cancer, it can be dealt with. What is essential is that she be given the facts in such a way that she can use them.

The unchanged rate of occurrence or incidence of breast cancer, 7 percent of all women of all ages, means several things. First and foremost, it means that 93 percent of women will not develop it. This is a remarkably large comfortable majority, all the warnings and crepe-hanging to the contrary. Second, it means that women today are no more likely to develop the cancer than were women twenty or forty years ago. This may seem strange in view of the talk on TV and in women's magazines about increased risks; about a woman, for example, who has her first baby after thirty, or a mother with cancer. The statistical phrase "at increased risk" means that such a woman is more likely to develop the cancer than a woman who lacks that particular experience or attribute, but we must examine these so-called risks. Like the actual percentage of women who do eventually get the cancer, those risks can be grossly exagger-

TABLE 1

CANCER OF THE BREAST IN WOMEN

Average annual age-specific incidence rates
per 100,000 population

AGE	INCIDENCE	PERCENTAGE OF WOMEN
15–19	——	——
20–24	1.1	0.001
25–29	8.7	0.009
30–34	22.5	0.02
35–39	52.5	0.05
40–44	103.7	0.10
45–49	159.2	0.16
50–54	171.7	0.17
55–59	191.8	0.19
60–64	226.2	0.23
65–69	234.2	0.23
70–74	259.8	0.26
75–79	294.9	0.30
80–84	301.3	0.30
85+	307.9	0.31

Incidence data from the Third National Cancer Survey; Incidence Data, National Institutes of Health, 1975. [2]

ated. Even though cancer of the breast is not increasing in frequency, we must admit that it is a potentially lethal cancer and that we must pay attention to it.

Looking at some other cancers that afflict women offers an informative perspective. Certain of these cancers are increasing in frequency; others, decreasing.[1] Lung cancer, due in large mea-

CHART 1

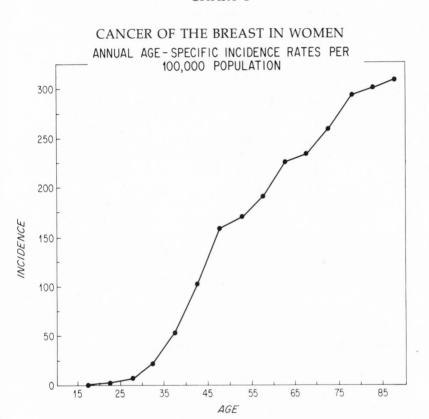

CANCER OF THE BREAST IN WOMEN
ANNUAL AGE-SPECIFIC INCIDENCE RATES PER
100,000 POPULATION

Incidence data from the Third National Cancer Survey; Incidence Data, National Institutes of Health, 1975.[2]

sure to smoking and other air pollutants, continues to increase in the male and has begun to increase in the female, a bad omen. The one measure we know to take is to give up smoking of tobacco, cigarettes in particular. Cancer of the stomach is decreasing as a problem, its incidence having gone down significantly. We do not know why. Control of cancer of the uterine cervix has improved enormously. Its occurrence is probably unchanged but the vaginal smear is picking it up in its initial phase before the malignant cells have begun to invade, when it is still *in situ* cancer and can be eradicated. The incidence of cancer of the lining of the uterus, like breast cancer, remains stable. Cancer of the ovary, on the other hand, is getting less and less frequent, almost disappearing.

A second fact important to our understanding is that the age at which breast cancer develops in women is also in essence unchanged. Although, as noted above, there is a suggestion that more younger women are now affected, the overall incidence rises in a straight line with increase in age.[2] Each year only 1 per 100,000 women aged 24 will be found to have the cancer. At age 30, 22 per 100,000, and at age 35, 52 per 100,000 will have developed it.* And 301 of the 100,000 who are aged 80 in any year will get it. (The age-specific incidence from 20 to 85 is given in Table 1 and Chart 1.[2]) Clearly, breast cancer is a disease of advancing age, but this is no reason for women to panic as they grow older. The 7 percent applies to all women, all ages included.

Let me repeat: considering the whole of her life, any one woman has only a 7 percent chance of getting breast cancer. If she is 30, the chance of her getting breast cancer that year is only 0.002 percent, since only 22 of 100,000 women of that age will get it. If she lives to 80 without getting the cancer, her chance of developing it in her 81st year has risen only to 0.3 percent (0.301 percent). Statistically, 301 women of 100,000 aged 80 will get it. As the statisticians put it, at age 80 the incidence is 301 cases per 100,000 women per annum.

These differences in the age in which breast cancer may be expected are important in regard to the diagnostic precautions that women should take. The precautions differ in degree and in

*These data from the National Cancer Institute of the age-specific incidence of breast cancer in women below the age of 35 may well be maximal. Data from Olmstead County, Minnesota, from 1945 to 1965 indicate a lesser incidence — two cancers per 100,000 women per annum in women 34 years or younger. Payne et al., *Arch. Surg.*, 101:105–113, 1970.

emphasis, becoming increasingly important with advancing age. This applies to the self-examination, the visits to doctors, mammographic x-rays, and so forth. These all become more important the longer one lives.

Other facts worthy of note are that breast cancer occurs in the male 100 times less frequently than in the female and that the incidence in the male also appears not to have changed.[1] The deductions are obvious. The preponderant incidence of breast cancer in the female must be related to the functional, hormonal, metabolic activity of the female breast. That the incidence in the male also has not changed over the last forty years suggests that no unusual influences affect the cancer in the male that do not also affect that in the female.

The stationary incidence of breast cancer in women over the last forty years is not only astounding; it is at first sight perplexing. We are hearing so much about women who are more likely than others to develop cancer, who are exceptional risks, who are said to be three times or seven times at greater risk than the average woman. There are many such reported risks: familial inherited risk, long ovarian life, use of estrogens, the Pill, fibrocystic changes, obesity, an underactive thyroid, and socioeconomic conditions.

If all of these risks are meaningful, why has the incidence of breast cancer not risen in the population? If the risks are meaningful, the incidence having remained stationary, then there must be individual women who are at lesser risk than others, women who are less likely than the average to develop cancer of the breast. There must be women who belong to groups of the population of whom only 1 or 2 percent will develop breast cancer. Who are all these women? What are the risks involved? Let us start with those risks that have been identified.

Familial-Genetic-Inherited Risk. Breast cancer is said to run in some families.[8–12] Yes, indeed, there are a number of instances where a mother, a daughter, and even a granddaughter develop breast cancer. Sometimes there is a mother, an aunt, and two daughters. Medical literature records instances in which as many as six or eight, though seldom more, women of a single family descending from a single grandmother have developed breast cancer. Such a family was first recorded by the French surgeon Paul Broca in 1866.[9]

Families with two or more members with breast cancer have been a special study of Dr. H. T. Lynch, of Omaha.[10,11] He and his colleagues have spent a lot of time ferreting out such families, searching the literature, following up reports from all over the country. Five years ago they had located thirty-four, and recently (1976) a total of fifty-two, such families. The history of one of these families is traced in Chart 5 of Dr. Lynch's 1972 article.[10]

But such families are rare. Dr. Lynch had a hard time finding the fifty-two. If the genetic influence were dominant, families like these ought to be all over the place. But they aren't. Also, if the influence were dominant, the number of cancer cases would be increasing. Yes, there must be some family-inherited influence, but it must be a recessive one. The number of families is small; the overall incidence of cancer has not increased in forty years. A woman whose mother or sister or aunt developed breast cancer does not need to feel she will "inherit" cancer or will have inherited a great risk of cancer. Yes, perhaps there is a small risk, but it is by no means positive that the daughter of a woman who had breast cancer will herself develop it. Think of the number of women with breast cancer whose daughters and granddaughters never develop the cancer. The vast majority of women who have breast cancer do not transmit the cancer to their offspring, or certainly not in a form in which the cancer eventually develops. The risk is slight but certainly slight only.

Certain Ovarian Histories. There are six conditions of women that appear statistically to influence the risk of breast cancer. A woman who has never had a child, or had her first baby after 30 or 35, or had an initial pregnancy at 18 or earlier, which was aborted — such a woman appears to have a somewhat greater incidence of breast cancer than the average woman.[8] On the other hand, a woman who had her first pregnancy before 18 (some say before 20), or who had her ovaries removed by the time she was 35 — that is, received a surgical menopause — is less likely to develop breast cancer than the average. Similarly, a woman who spontaneously had a short ovarian life without intervention — that is, a late onset of her periods, at 16 or 18 (late menarche), and an early menopause, before 40 — is less prone to the cancer.

Use of Estrogens. The taking of estrogens, the female sex hormone, in one form or another is believed by many to influence the occurrence of breast and uterine cancers.[3,13–18] Such suspicion is reasonable, since estrogens are a normal stimulant of both the breasts and the uterus, and given in pill form they increase the amount within the body. If the dose is more than minimal, it increases the thickening and lumpiness of the breast and brings about abnormal bleeding from the uterus.

But if estrogens are truly a cause of breast cancer, it is surprising that the incidence of the cancer has not risen sharply in the last fifteen years in the United States. In the past twenty-five years, a growing number of American women have been taking estrogens for one reason or another. Many gynecologists routinely place their patients on estrogens after a hysterectomy, and hysterectomy has been and still is a common operation.

Women have also been advised to take the female hormone to stay young.[15] Others take it in lesser doses to avoid hot flashes of the menopause, and some to prevent thinning of the bones (osteoporosis). It is estimated by the drug houses who sell the hormones that twenty million women have been taking estrogens in the last ten years. If estrogens were an important cause of breast cancer, surely the incidence of the cancer should be increasing, and as yet this does not appear to be so.

Cancers of the lining of the uterus, however, are believed to have increased over the last five years in women taking estrogen pills.[17,18] It may be that the lining of the uterus, the endometrium, is more susceptible than the tissues of the breast.

Experience with an especially potent chemically synthesized

estrogen, diethylstilbesterol, suggests that there may indeed be a difference in the sensitivity of the breast compared with the uterus and other tissues of woman.[19] In the years immediately after World War II many physicians throughout the United States prescribed this substance (DES) for pregnant women who had hemorrhaged or miscarried in a previous pregnancy. The pregnancies fared well, apparently. By 1970, however, a few of the daughters in their late teens and early twenties were found to have developed a special type of cancer of the vagina and cervix. This finding was immediately alarming because it is a rare cancer and almost never encountered in a young woman of 20. It was postulated that the cancer had resulted from premature stimulation by the hormone of the fetus's vagina and uterine cervix during their development in the mother's uterus.

There has been a great scare about this cancer and other possible complications in the children, both daughters and sons, of mothers who had been so treated. Fortunately this reality is proving to be less bad than feared at first. At latest reports only 330 daughters of between two and three million children have developed the vaginal and cervical cancer. In many other young women signs of an overstimulated vaginal and uterine lining were found, but these signs are gradually disappearing. None of the breasts of the daughters have been adversely affected, suggesting a lesser sensitivity of their breasts to this hormone during fetal life. Although the testes of some of the sons are smaller than the expected average size, and their sperm appear slightly abnormal, none of the sons has developed a cancer and none is proven sterile. Even though the number of children affected is less than feared, all the children, particularly the daughters, should, until the scare is past, report to one of the special clinics that have been organized by the National Cancer Institute for their watchful care. Parents, daughters, and sons who wish additional information and the address of the special follow-up clinics should write to the Office of Cancer Communication, National Cancer Institute, National Institutes of Health, Bethesda, Maryland 20014.

It is to be emphasized that this experience with diethylstilbesterol is numerically a limited one.[19] The hormone was used for this purpose for a very short period only, and was given up long ago. I mention the experience partly as a warning but principally to give comfort to those women who have been taking estrogens in lesser doses for reasons other than preventing miscarriage.

The Pill. The Pill as a possible hazard has raised a special question.[20,21] Some women with active fibrocystic changes have been relieved of the pain in their breasts by going on the Pill. In some, the lumpiness of the changes has been decreased. The Pill, instead of a hazard, may be a good treatment for women whose breasts have developed the fibrocystic disorder.

Fibrocystic Changes. It is said that women who have had fibrocystic disease are at special risk in developing breast cancer; that is, they are more likely to develop the cancer than those women who never had the fibrocystic disorder.[22,23] Specifically, it is reported by some statisticians that a woman who has had a breast cyst has three times the risk of developing the cancer. How do they know there is an increased risk and how can they be sure it is three and not some other number? What are the facts, if there are any, behind such statements?

First, fibrocystic changes are a common disorder affecting a majority of women in the United States. (Virginia Frantz and her colleagues found it in 53 percent of 225 women whose breasts were examined at autopsy.[24])

Second, the disorder is almost certainly on the increase because of birth control. Pregnancy absorbs the changes, and the decrease in the number of pregnancies from three or more to two or fewer has an inevitable influence.

Third, nobody knows how many women, certainly a minority, never have these changes.

Fourth, because more women now have these changes, the incidence of breast cancer should have increased if the changes are truly a contributing cause of the cancer. But breast cancer has not increased.

Fifth, since nobody knows the number or proportion of

women who have never had fibrocystic changes, nobody can compare the incidence of cancer between those who have and those who have not had these changes. The phrase "three times at risk," therefore, has no basis and is meaningless.

Recently I was consulted by a woman of 42 from a major New England city. Two breast cysts had been resected; one, two years before, the other, two years earlier. Now she had a third cyst. Her surgeon and his hospital's oncologist (both men and both on the faculty of the local medical school) told her that, because of the cysts, she was "three times at risk." They advised her, therefore, to avoid cancer by having both breasts removed. She had two well children, 20 and 18 years old. She had separated from her husband because of his attentions to other women and was about to start divorce proceedings. She was making her own living as a remedial teacher. She hoped some day to find another man with whom she would have a more congenial marriage. What thoughtless, insensitive advice to give to any woman, and certainly a woman in her circumstances. And on what basis, what facts? When she asked, her doctors told her they were following the advice of the cancer authorities, the American Cancer Society.

Are her doctors to blame or are the professionals of the cancer centers? What a loose, irresponsible claim "three times at risk" can be. Women should insist on a detailed, factual analysis of statements regarding risks. Too often the statements are careless, and sometimes unjustified. The facts usually dissipate much of the anxiety.

The most one can say is that the breast, if subjected to hormone stimulation uninterrupted by pregnancies, may provide a more fertile ground in which a cancer subsequently may grow.

Obesity. Fat women are more likely to develop breast cancer than the thin.[25] This is a statistical fact. It is, however, not clear why this should be so. Some believe it is because fat cells have the ability to change the male sex hormone circulating in the woman into the female hormone, and the fat woman in reality has an excessive amount of female hormone. The risk is slight, and there are other reasons to avoid being fat, more important than the possible increased risk of breast cancer. Fat people often suffer high blood pressure, difficulties with cardiac and liver functions, diabetes, and other problems. It's best to avoid unnecessary overweight for all of them.

Hypothyroidism. Women whose thyroid function is reduced for one reason or another are more prone to develop breast cancer than are normal women.[25–28] Recent analyses of the prolactin- and thyroid-stimulating hormones indicate that there is an overlap in their secretion, and that the body's urge to stimulate the thyroid gland to produce more hormone has a comparable effect on the prolactin secretion; the slightly greater cancer risk comes from the prolactin. Patients with reduced or absent thyroid function need medication for their general health. Attending to the thyroid need itself does away with the added risk.

X-Rays. The medical profession and the public are currently much worried about unnecessary use of x-rays, particularly in young people. X-ray treatment around the head and neck, given for acne of the face or for tonsillitis or for other reasons, has resulted ten to twenty years later in a slightly increased incidence of papillary goiter, a sluggish type of malignancy. X-ray of other tissues in young people has also occasionally induced a malignant degeneration, and the profession is wary of possible injury to the breast caused by the taking of too many mammograms.[29–31] X-ray penetration is necessary to obtain a picture of the breast. No breast malignancy has as yet been recorded from the taking of mammograms. Nobody knows what the dangerous dose is. It is likely to be age-related. Later we will lay down rules regarding the taking of x-ray pictures of the breast. It's a risk, but not a great one. There are benefits that transcend the risk.

Socioeconomic Conditions. The socioeconomic condition of people apparently does affect the incidence of breast cancer.[32] The disease is encountered more frequently in those who live under more privileged circumstances. The reason for this is not understood. Whatever the stimulus, it is not great, and those who are less well-off are not at significant advantage as far as the development of breast cancer is concerned.

Of No Moment. Women are constantly asking whether there is anything about their diet, lovemaking that involves the breast, trauma, and the place or climate they live in that predisposes them to breast cancer. Aside from a diet that is conducive to obesity, there is no known diet that leads to breast cancer or makes a woman less susceptible. Prolonged breast fondling or suckling theoretically might activate lactation but it presumably should not induce cancer. Trauma, as we have already said, is not a cause.

Geography and Climate. The incidence of breast cancer appears to be unaffected by climate or geography per se in the United States.[2,3]

Religious Groups. Those special circumstances that are associated with certain religious groups are reported to lower slightly the incidence of breast cancer.[33,34] There is reportedly less breast cancer among women members of the Seventh Day Adventist and Mormon churches than among women living in the same geographical area who are not members of those churches. The reasons for this have not been identified.

I have gone into aspects of the incidence and risks of developing breast cancer in such detail to make sure that you women, my readers, will understand why I think too much alarm over "risks" has been raised in the last ten years by many physicians and surgeons, the American Cancer Society, and, more recently, by officials of the National Cancer Institute. Much of what has been said and is being said is exaggerated, unclear, and therefore misleading and thoughtless of women. The majority of statements are made by physicians and epidemiologists who are overly concerned with their corner of expertise and are not thinking of the human concerns of women, the women who must bear the brunt — all the benign troubles, the fears, and the cancers as well.

One question: of all the physicians, doctors, and epidemiologists, how many are women? Almost none.

Only 7 percent of all women in the U.S.A. are going to have breast cancer; 93 percent of women are not.

Improvements in our knowledge will bring this 7 percent down as current research increases our understanding and improves our care.

Then there are other reasons why women should worry less about breast cancer. New knowledge is not the only thing forthcoming. As we shall see in the following chapters, the old treatments, unsatisfactory for so many women, are giving way to new methods, new approaches, with new hope.

Chapter 6

Surgery — The First Hope

IT IS ALMOST IMPOSSIBLE for those of us living in the latter half of the twentieth century to visualize what cancer of the breast meant to women living before the development of modern surgery. Until the discovery of anesthesia in 1846 and the understanding and control of wound infection thirty years later, treatment was virtually no better in the first half of the nineteenth century than it had been in ancient times — salves and liniments for ulcerations, brutal excision of the breast by cautery or scalpel, treatments totally inadequate to deal with the painful ulcerated tumors of the chest wall and slow destruction of the vital liver, lungs, and bones. Cancer of the breast was a scourge, one of the most horrible.

The advent of modern surgery changed all this. The discovery of anesthesia made it possible for a woman to bear a long operation.[1] With care and finesse, the surgeon could then cut away the cancerous breast and many of the lymph nodes to which the cancer might have spread. The realization by Joseph Lister that bacteria, discovered by Louis Pasteur, were the probable cause of wound infection and gangrene made surgical care not only endurable but feasible.[2] The coming of modern surgery was a boon to the woman with breast cancer.

At this writing, most doctors and surgeons in this country agree that surgery is the primary therapy of breast cancer, and radical mastectomy the operation of choice. For eighty-one years it has remained the standard for treatment. What is more, the American Cancer Society recommends radical mastectomy (or its variant, the modified radical) as the *only* tried, and therefore the *only* acceptable, treatment.[3] Before we look once again at what this operation accomplishes and what it does to the woman who undergoes it, let us examine anatomically what it is and how it came about.[4]

William Stewart Halsted described the removal of the entire breast containing the cancer, the lymph nodes of the axilla to which the cancer might have spread, and the major pectoral muscle, which lies between breast and axilla, interfering with the surgeon's approach to the axillary nodes. The smaller pectoral muscle (*pectoralis minor*) was severed at one end and retracted to open the access to the nodes. The nipple and the major portion of the skin over the breast were removed. Only enough skin on the sides of the breast was left to bring the edges of the skin together and thus close the wound over the chest wall. The resulting scar of the operation ran from the front of the upper arm down across the shoulder joint, down the front of the chest over the defect where the pectoral muscle had been, and along the line where the nipple had been to the bottom crease of the breast. All of the fat beneath the skin was scrupulously removed, together with the thin fibrous sheath overlying the ribs and the rib muscles. The unexcised skin, closed over the defect where the breast and muscle had been, lay flat against the chest wall, tight and motionless. To get rid of the primary tumor, the breast was removed. To get all of the nodes of the axilla, the muscle was removed. The removal of both left not only a hideous defect in the upper chest, but a significant handicap to the motion of the arm as well.

The operation was also frequently followed by pain since it cut across many sensory nerves. This we learned from the experience of the third patient described in Chapter 2. Furthermore, with the removal of the highest nodes of the axilla, the lymph flow from the arm is always blocked to an extent and some swelling of the arm is common.

Halsted was insistent that the breast, the axillary fat containing the lymph nodes, and the intervening muscle be excised all in one piece, and that at no point should the surgeon cut into a cancerous area, for fear of releasing a cancer-inciting chemical or disseminating malignant cells with the scalpel. He also held, and for the same reasons, that the surgeon should not cut into the tumor for biopsy at the beginning of the operation. The surgeon should, in Halsted's opinion, be sufficiently versed in the clinical nature of the disease to be able to make the diagnosis without the preliminary biopsy and help of the pathologist. (He was later to change his mind about these needs.)

Halsted was by no means alone in seeking to find the best possible operation for relief of breast cancer. Many surgeons of the Western world — in Europe, the British Isles, Canada, and the United States — tried and described various procedures in the twenty years before Halsted's paper appeared. Halsted was aware of the work of several German surgeons who found it important (as did some English surgeons) to remove the lymph nodes of the axilla as well as the breast. They had also found it necessary to remove the pectoral muscles in order to obtain a proper surgical view of the armpit. He was particularly impressed with Richard von Volkmann's meticulous resection of the fine fascial layer (the thin sheet of fibrous tissue) overlying the chest wall, but felt Volkmann did not pursue the excision far enough.[5] And in the United States, he felt that the famous Philadelphia surgeons Samuel David Gross and David Hayes Agnew, who claimed that breast cancer was incurable, were unnecessarily pessimistic. Most surprising of all, in the very year that Halsted's paper appeared, 1894, Willie Meyer, of New York, was practicing in essence the same operation as Halsted.[6] How is it, then, that after so much study and effort by others, Halsted should have received the world's acclaim and credit for the operation?

Halsted did far more than describe an operative procedure. He laid down the principles of the so-called follow-up, by which doctors were to keep track of patients for months or years to determine whether they had been cured by the operation. If a surgeon of the time repaired a hernia or removed stones from the gall bladder, he felt the patient was cured once the wound had healed. Too often the surgeon assumed that if the patient with breast cancer left the hospital with the wound free of infection, the edges of the skin together and healing well, and with no gross evidence of any cancer, she too was cured. But this was not so with cancer of the breast. Before long, patients would reappear with cancer growing again, either in the wound of the chest or elsewhere in the body. Surgeons differed in their opinions as to what this meant. Albert Billroth, the famous surgeon of Austria, felt that if there was no reappearance of the cancer within a year, the patient was cured; if cancer reappeared a year and a half after operation, it must be a new cancer.[7]

Halsted differed with this point of view. If the cancer reappeared within three years, it must be the same cancer. If the patient lived on well for three years, time enough had elapsed for the patient to be considered cured of the disease.

From 1889 to 1894 Halsted performed radical mastectomies on fifty women with cancer of the breast. In his aftercare of the patients, he set an example. He followed them as meticulously as he had done the operation. Seeing them at frequent and regular intervals, he knew just how they fared. He described their course in detail in his paper of 1894. Such aftercare was then a rarity.

In the next several years he realized that three years was not long enough to assume that the patient was cured even if no cancer had reappeared. Patients were returning after more than three years with cancer growing once again in the wound or elsewhere, and he had reason to know it must be the same cancer, not a new one. How he came to know this is in itself illustrative of his extraordinary care. After removing a breast and its cancer he would depart from the operating table with the specimen, leaving his assistants to sew up the wound. He would then study the cancer in detail, marking special pieces with silk ties for later study under the microscope.[8] In this manner he came to know the several types of cancer, and when a cancer nodule appeared in the mastectomy wound he could distinguish a regrowth of the original cancer from a new cancer. By 1907, when he made his second report, now having operated on 232 patients, he realized that a five-year follow-up was necessary.[9]

Because of his painstaking care of the patients and the detailed reporting of the results, his influence held sway. From 1907 to this day, five-year follow-up has remained the standard by which most physicians measure the success of the operation. As we shall see later, this five-year follow-up, reasonable seventy years ago, is no longer a tenable period by which to judge the effectiveness of an operation in a disease as variable in its behavior as cancer of the breast.

The repeated recurrence of the cancer in the wound area of some patients, the continued death of some before the fifth year, and the death of many more from the cancer after five years led inevitably to a search for methods of improving the operation. Surgery was the only therapy of any use, and surgeons clung to the concept that if they could but improve the operative technique, more and more patients would be relieved and cured.

Halsted was himself one of the first to seek better ways of performing his operation. He extended the excision of lymph nodes to include those at the base of the neck above the clavicle.[8] This procedure he later abandoned because he soon realized that these nodes were involved only after prolonged involvement of the axillary nodes. He also excised more widely the skin of the breast, leaving a gap between the skin flaps. This defect he closed with a graft of skin from the thigh or elsewhere.[10] He continued painstakingly to follow all his patients and to seek all avenues of getting patients to report earlier in the course of their disease, when the chance of cure was better.

In 1912, Sampson Handley, of the Middlesex Hospital in London, reported the resection of lymph nodes from under the breastbone (the sternum), the so-called internal mammary nodes.[11] Halsted in his original paper had described three patients from whom Harvey Cushing, his resident at the time, had resected cancerous tissue from the chest wall, tissue apparently emanating from the lymph nodes beneath the sternum.[4] But, curiously, Halsted paid no further attention to this observation of Cushing's. Handley, on the other hand, pursued the matter, found that these nodes were not uncommonly involved, and devised an operation to remove them as well as those of the axilla. The new operation did not improve the results, and he soon abandoned it. Many years later, after World War II, this same effort was taken up by Jerome Urban of the Memorial Hospital in New York and E. Dahl-Iversen and T. Tobiassen of Copenhagen.[12,13] The operation was a massive, disabling one; it called for resecting the rib cartilages at the side of the sternum and excising the involved lymph nodes beneath. The operation, known as the extended radical or the super-radical mastectomy, was practiced until very recently, but has now been abandoned by most surgeons because it brought no better results than the standard traditional Halsted mastectomy.

Other efforts at improving the cure rate have included removal of the other breast to eliminate the possibility of a second cancer, and adding a small dose of irradiation to kill any cancer cells left in the field of operation. As we shall see, these two measures have also not materially altered the outcome.

These efforts were all directed to improving the radical mastectomy operation. Departures from the traditional operation were slow to come. The first departure of note was made by Geoffrey Keynes, at St. Bartholomew's Hospital in London, starting in 1924.[14] He recognized that the cure rate after radical mastectomy was significantly lower than anticipated. Radium and x-ray had become available, and at his professor's suggestion, Keynes undertook a trial of radiation. At first he used radium and x-ray in conjunction with the operation. Then he found he could achieve the same result by combining radiation with the removal of just the tumor rather than the whole breast. There followed several reports advocating the use of radiation.

In this country, Leland McKittrick, in Boston, followed his example, using radium to supplement radical mastectomy. Keynes and McKittrick reported together, in 1937, before the American Surgical Association.[15,16] The results of adding radium to the operation unfortunately did not improve the outcome, and almost nobody followed suit in this country.

Keynes, in contrast, became increasingly interested in irradiation as an alternative to radical mastectomy, and the number of patients who were so treated increased. Keynes's results were questioned by many, and in 1948 Sir James Patterson Ross, then the professor of surgery at St. Bartholomew's Hospital, reviewed Keynes's fifteen years of work.[17] The results of irradiation alone were indeed the equal of those in patients treated over the same period at the same hospital by radical mastectomy. Ross also found that the results compared favorably with two separate series of patients treated by radical mastectomy by two prominent surgeons at two other London hospitals. Irradiation, thus proven to have a place as an alternative treatment, was still considered not more successful than radical mastectomy.

In Scotland during World War II, R. McWhirter, a radiologist at Edinburgh, trained at St. Bartholomew's Hospital before the war during the time of Keynes, tried the simpler surgical procedure of removing only the breast, following it by radiation of the axillary lymph nodes.[18] His results, though disputed by most American surgeons, appeared to be the equal of the radical operation. Even more recently, several surgeons, recognizing the disability to the arm resulting from the excision of the muscles, have been preserving the muscles, reaching up under them as high as possible, getting most, but not necessarily all, of the nodes.[19,20] And now, recent evidence indicates that this simpler procedure, called the modified radical, is followed by results the equal of those of the traditional radical.[21]

The development of the radical mastectomy in the 1890s, so early in the years of modern surgery, was in itself an achievement. That Halsted should have attempted to measure its success in his painstaking follow-up was equally important. Halsted was an unusually thoughtful, imaginative, innovative person. He was perhaps the more interesting because during this phase of his life he had become addicted to cocaine. Some have thought that his struggle with the addiction was in some measure responsible for his meticulous attention to details and for his innovative scholarship.[22] His full story is yet to be unfolded but certain it is that he was a man of remarkable character and influence, and these personal qualities were a substantial reason why so much attention was paid to his operation.[23] Addicted or not to cocaine or morphine or both, his accomplishments were prodigious, and he impressed all who came to study under him.

The story of the surgical treatment of breast cancer is, in its way, a glorious one. Surgery came on the scene when there was no other treatment of note. It brought relief and hope. Still useful in a limited way, still needed to help establish the diagnosis, major surgery as therapy has had its day. Mastectomy in any of its forms is on its way out.

By what authority do I say that? What right have I to say it? What is the evidence for so sweeping a conclusion? Before presenting the evidence, I shall say something of my personal experience and my right to speak.

I am just old enough to have seen patients with advanced neglected cancer of the breast. As a fourth-year medical student, in the summer of 1927, I went into the back country of Rhode Island to pay a visit to an old farmer-friend and his wife. He had taught me as a boy how to pitch hay and load a hay wagon. He was well, but she was confined upstairs. She called to me from the window, asking me to come up and see her. She had a big ulcerating tumor in one of her breasts, and, almost certainly, metastases in her bones. The local physician had died several months earlier, but because I was a medical student, she thought of me as a doctor and asked for my advice. All I could do was to get her to the hospital in Providence, where she died shortly thereafter. From that time on, I have been caring for patients with breast cancer, caring for them with the advice and help of many colleagues, older and younger. As an intern and resident, from 1928 through 1932, I was schooled in the performance of a radical mastectomy by two of Boston's foremost surgeons, Drs. E. P. Richardson and E. D. Churchill, both professors of surgery at the Harvard Medical School and chiefs of surgical services at the Massachusetts General Hospital. Churchill was particularly imbued with Halsted's meticulous technique, and he taught me the importance of securing each little vessel so that when the skin was sewn together, the wound beneath did not seep and did not need to be drained. The wound without drains tended to be more comfortable than one with drains, and the likelihood of infection was reduced. Because this was a period of training, I concentrated on the techniques needed to become expert. I accepted the traditional thinking and asked no questions.

In 1937 I was assigned to deliver the formal lectures on diseases of the breast to the students of the Harvard Medical School. Such an assignment was a prize for a young surgeon. I realized that it was given to me because of my interest in endocrinology and that I was expected to look at breast diseases from the point of view of hormone changes. It was a new point of view for the time, and the assignment proved a step forward in my education. I saw how the breast and uterus responded in parallel fashion to the same ovarian hormones, and how comparable were the diseases of the two organs. For drawing this analogy, I got a lot of flak from the gynecologists and the pathologists, but it has come to be accepted now, and this is the background, of course, for what I have written about fibrocystic disease.

Open-minded about the functional, hormonal troubles of the breast, I was blind to the problems of cancer. I accepted what I had been told. I kept on doing the traditional radical mastectomy through the time of treating and following up the three patients of 1943, described in Chapter 2. I was brought up short by the mutilation and cruelty of losing a breast suffered by each of those patients. Equally important, these women made me realize how little I knew about the disease of breast cancer. Still, I went on doing radical mastectomies for each patient with breast cancer until 1956. Then, for the first time, I met a patient who refused to have a mastectomy. It was not that she was afraid of an operation — she had asked me to operate on her goiter — but she was adamant about her breast, and I had to arrange an alternative for her. She allowed me to resect just the tumor, and Dr. L. L. Robbins, chief of our radiology department, undertook to irradiate the remainder of her breast, and she was gratified.

Then, in 1958, the widow of one of my teachers of medicine refused to have a mastectomy in any form, and told me why. She made me look at the cruelty of my trade, the surgeon's trade. The cruelty was particularly clear when I realized that radiation following a limited surgical excision could provide an alternative as it had in the patient of two years before. I have recounted her experiences in two articles (*Radcliffe Quarterly*, 1970,[24] and *Psychiatry in Medicine*, 1971[25]), and I shall talk more about her in Chapter 11. It was she who forced me finally to look critically at the operation of radical mastectomy to see just what it was accomplishing. I had to ask myself three questions. Was I justified in acquiescing to her demand to provide her with a less mutilating treatment? Had I harmed the earlier patient? And should I have found a way to convince both patients to accept the mastectomy? There was now no escape; I had to examine what radical mastectomy really amounted to. As I looked, the evidence against the operation was convincing; so convincing, indeed, that I did my last radical mastectomy in 1960.

The years since 1956 have shown me only the more clearly that mastectomy has not lived up to expectations, that it cures but the minority, that the results have not improved over the last forty years, that it is long outdated and is to be superseded. The evidence for the low cure rate and lack of improvement is based on statistical data, and I shall present the data in historical sequence. Now to the statistics.

In order to examine the effectiveness of an operation, one must know first what happens to patients who receive no treatment whatsoever, and compare their course with that of patients who are operated on. For the purpose of this comparison there are, unfortunately, only three reports in the world medical literature of what happens to patients who receive no treatment. The first is an account from the Middlesex Hospital in London over the 100-year period from 1820 to 1920.[26] For the most part it was a period when there was no treatment, and patients came only when they were in a difficult state, late in the course of the disease. The life history of the disease in these patients was therefore hard to reconstruct. There are only two accounts of patients in the twentieth century, in more modern times when the surgical operation had been perfected and a modern therapy was available. The first was a report by Ernest Daland, in 1927, of 100 patients, encountered in Harvard cancer hospitals, who had received no treatment.[27] Eight years later approximately half of

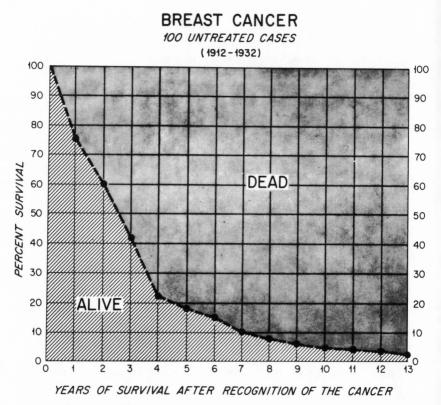

BREAST CANCER
100 UNTREATED CASES
(1912-1932)

YEARS OF SURVIVAL AFTER RECOGNITION OF THE CANCER

Fig. 1: *The life course of 100 patients with untreated breast cancer. All patients to the right of the curve are dead (shaded area), whereas those to the left of the curve are still alive (striped area). Data redrawn from Nathanson and Welch (1937).*[28]

these same patients, with another 50 added, were recorded by Ira Nathanson and Claude Welch.[28] The course of the lives of these 100 patients is shown graphically in Figure 1. The length of time these patients lived after the tumor was first recognized varied considerably. The majority of the patients died in the early

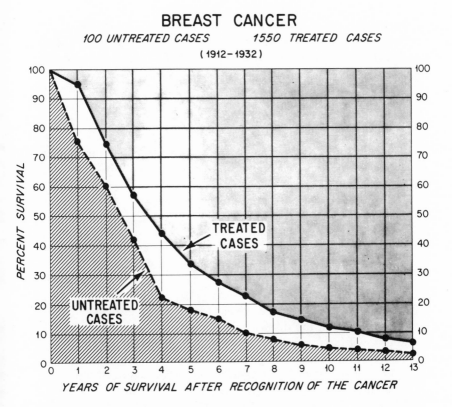

Fig. 2: *The life course of 1550 patients treated by radical mastectomy (1912 to 1932) compared with that of the 100 untreated patients shown in Fig. 1. Data redrawn from Nathanson and Welch (1937).*[28]

years but others survived for eight and ten years, and two were still alive at the end of the study in the thirteenth year. It is clearly a disease of great variability.

Nathanson and Welch then compared the survival period of these 100 untreated patients with that of 1550 patients who had been treated at the same time in the same Harvard hospitals by radical mastectomy. The course of these 1550 patients is shown in Figure 2, together with those of the 100 untreated. The difference between the curves of the untreated and treated indicates that the survival of many of those treated was a little longer in the initial years after operation. In the period from the fourth to the sixth year after operation, the treated patients survived two years longer than the untreated. And this longer survival remained for the next few years through the eleventh year. But as more and more patients who had been operated upon died, by the thirteenth year there was little difference between the two — only 6 percent of the operated patients were still alive, 94 percent having died, presumably of their cancer. The only conclusion possible was that operation postponed death from the disease; true cures were few.

The second way of examining the effectiveness of an operation is by following a substantial number of patients through their lives, plotting the time when deaths occur, and measuring the survival of the remainder for a period long enough to be reasonably sure that they have been cured of the cancer. We saw that from 1900 to 1920 five years was considered a sufficiently long period. Then it was realized five years was not long enough, and ten years was selected. Subsequently, it has become clear that the disease may be even slower to take its toll, and now fifteen years is considered the minimum time by which cure can be claimed.

One of the first to plot the number of years that patients survive radical mastectomy was Stuart Harrington of the Mayo Clinic (1953).[29] He showed the survival rate of more than 4500 patients for fifteen to forty years following radical mastectomy (Table 2). Only one quarter of the patients lived for as long as fifteen years. Harrington presumed that the 75 percent who

TABLE 2.†

UNILATERAL CARCINOMA OF THE BREAST (FEMALES): SURVIVAL RATES 15 TO 40 YEARS FOLLOWING RADICAL MASTECTOMY.

| | PATIENTS | | LIVED INDICATED PERIOD | |
YEARS POST-OPERATIVE	TOTAL	TRACED	NUMBER	PER-CENTAGE*
15 or more	4637	4563 (98.4%)	1144	25.1
20 or more	3615	3544 (98.0%)	624	17.6
25 or more	2439	2391 (98.0%)	301	12.6
30 or more	1415	1375 (97.2%)	128	9.3
35 to 40	520	507 (97.5%)	35	6.6

Based on traced patients. Inquiry as of January 1, 1950.
†*Copy of original table, Harrington, 1953.* [29]

were known to have died in those fifteen years had died of their cancer.

The first comprehensive account of the ultimate results of various forms of mastectomy, with or without radiation, came in 1953, from St. Bartholomew's Hospital in London. Dr. I. G. Williams, director of radiotherapy, Mr. R. S. Murley, a surgeon, and Mr. M. P. Curwen, a medical statistician, reported the course of life of 1044 patients treated from 1930 through 1952.[30] Nearly half received a radical mastectomy; a lesser number, a modified radical operation (the pectoral muscles were not excised); and the remaining minority, a simple excision plus irradiation. There was no significant difference in outcome among the three treatments. The results of the entire series are depicted in a single graph, Figure 3. The graph is a model presentation of such cancer mortality data, and the following are to be noted.

Depicted at the top is the number of patients lost track of dur-

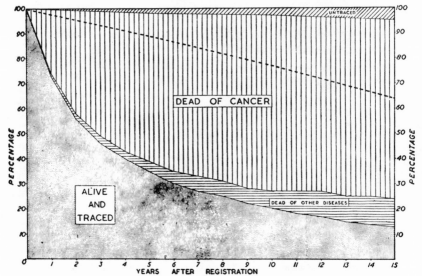

Percentages dead and alive based on whole series (1–15 years). (The dotted line indicates the expected survival of a normal group with similar age distribution based on Life Table for 1931.)

Fig. 3: *A photographic reproduction of the figure in the paper by Williams et al., with its original legend from St. Bartholomew's Hospital, London, 1953.*[30]

ing the study — 5 percent. Lower in the graph is the number of those who died of other causes — 11 percent. The obvious and appalling fact found was that 75 percent of the patients had died of the cancer despite treatment, and only 13 percent of the patients were alive at the end of the fifteenth year. Almost no attention has been paid either to Harrington's report or to this one, both of 1953. Yet since 1965 the findings have been confirmed repeatedly in England, the United States, and Canada.

Statisticians have pointed out that it is not fair to ascribe all of the deaths in Table 2 to cancer of the breast. It is quite possible that some of the women might have died of heart attacks,

pneumonia, or from automobile accidents, troubles quite unre-
lated to the breast cancer. Williams and his colleagues obviously
dealt with this problem in their 1953 report by eliminating from
the cancer deaths those who died of other causes. Clearly, accurate recording of the cause of death was needed. Except for
Williams, few have made such information available.

This reservation of the statisticians is of course correct. As we
shall see, it applies to a valid but complicated statistical problem
dealt with differently by various physicians. Death from other
causes is not the only correction that should be applied. If the
effectiveness of the operation in curing the cancer is at issue,
then it is essential to know if residual cancer was present in the
patient dying of an automobile accident or other noncancer
cause. All of the patients had breast cancer to begin with, and
because the cancer carries such a high mortality despite surgical
mastectomy or other local treatment, a patient who died of a
heart attack or automobile accident may well have had, hidden
deep in the body, residual cancer that eventually would have
killed her. So to be fair in judging the usefulness of the operation, a correction would have to be made in the opposite direction. But what is the amount of the correction to be made? In
many instances neither the cause of death nor the presence of
residual cancer is known with certainty. Such information
would require either complete physician's notes regarding the
condition of the patient immediately before death or an autopsy
in which residual cancer was looked for. Since notes of this sort
and autopsy reports have been available in only a minority of patients in the United States, many physicians think that death
curves should not be corrected either for the noncancer deaths
or for probable residual cancer. Increasingly, cancer statistics are
being gathered in registries, where physicians' opinions as well
as postmortem examinations are carefully correlated. Future
cancer statistics both in this country and abroad will therefore
portray the reality more and more closely.

Since 1966 several reports have appeared in England, Canada,
and the United States supporting the results recorded by Harrington and by Williams and his co-workers in 1953. In some of

TABLE 3
LONG-TERM SURVIVAL FOLLOWING THREE METHODS OF TREATMENT

AUTHORS	NUMBER PATIENTS	PERCENT SURVIVAL — YEARS				REMARKS
		5	10	15	20	
SURVIVAL FOLLOWING RADICAL MASTECTOMY						
1. Berg, Robbins, 1966[31]	1,458	62	50	43	40	
2. McLaughlin, Coe, 1969[32]	292	62	26	13	3	
3. Peters, 1970[33]	2,316	60	40	27	19	Radical mastectomy plus radiation
	219	60	31	20	9	Radical mastectomy only
4. Cutler, Heise, 1971[34]	13,274	53	40	34	30	1940–1949 Series
	Not given	60	48	41	(36)*	1950–1954 Series
	15,653	63	(50)*	(43)*	(39)*	1960–1964 Series
		*( ) = Calculated				
5. Lee, Lambley, 1971[35]	230	—	49	35	—	
6. Campos, 1972[36]	184	80	61	50	—	Negative Nodes
7. Ruiz, et al., 1973[37]	394	—	24	10	2	
SURVIVAL FOLLOWING SIMPLE MASTECTOMY AND IRRADIATION						
8. Bruce, 1971[32]	413	58	39	31	—	
SURVIVAL FOLLOWING LUMPECTOMY AND PRIMARY IRRADIATION						
9. Peters, 1970[33]	80	60	28	14	13	
10. Mustakallio, 1972[38]	702	80	60	47	—	

the reports the statistics have been corrected for life expectancy of people of the same age; in others, not. In none of the corrected reports was the probable continued presence of cancer considered. Since residual cancer was presumably present in at least 50 percent of the patients dying from other causes, the corrected curves for the effectiveness of radical mastectomy in curing the cancer were overcorrected.

The data and the authors of seven of these modern reports are given in Table 3.* A composite graph of five of them appears in Figure 4. The graph depicts the survival (or the reverse, the mortality) of several thousand women with cancer of the breast treated by radical mastectomy and followed for fifteen to twenty years. The data corrected for life expectancy are shown with broken lines; uncorrected data, with solid lines. The uniform downward trend of these curves is striking, and the data provide unchallengeable support for the statement that the majority of patients with breast cancer ultimately succumb to the cancer despite the operation of radical mastectomy. Let us examine these more modern data in detail.

All show fewer than 50 percent of the patients alive by the fifteenth year. The best results (or the least bad) are those corrected for life expectancy, and the best of these indicate that only 48 percent of the patients were alive fifteen years after mastectomy. The results in the uncorrected series are generally lower and the average is nearer 25 percent survival at fifteen years. The lowest curve depicts a most carefully followed series of 292 patients operated upon by Dr. Charles McLaughlin, recent past president of the American College of Surgeons.[32] He knew the cause of death in all of his patients; almost all of the deaths were due to the cancer. Only thirteen of the patients were alive at fifteen years and only three at twenty years. Knowing his careful technique, we can only judge that it was not lack of skill or of care but rather the nature of the disease that thwarted Dr. McLaughlin's efforts to cure more of the patients.

The uniformity of the results at fifteen years after radical mas-

*The references for the articles are given in the notes for this chapter, for those wishing to examine the data in detail.[31–37]

RADICAL MASTECTOMY

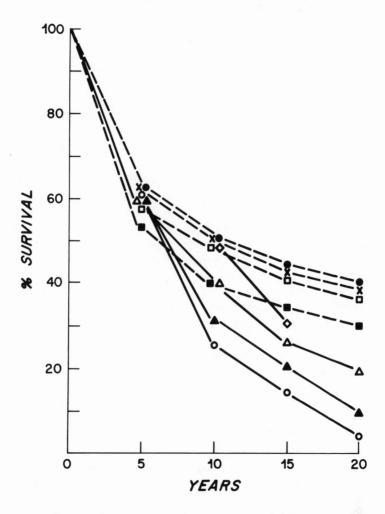

Fig. 4: *Percent survival after radical mastectomy — 15-to-20-year follow-up. The survival curves corrected for life expectancy are depicted with broken lines (Berg and Robbins,*[31] *Cutler and Heise*[34]*). Uncorrected with solid lines (McLaughlin and Coe,*[32] *Peters,*[33] *Lee and Lambley*[35]*).*

MASTECTOMY & IRRADIATION

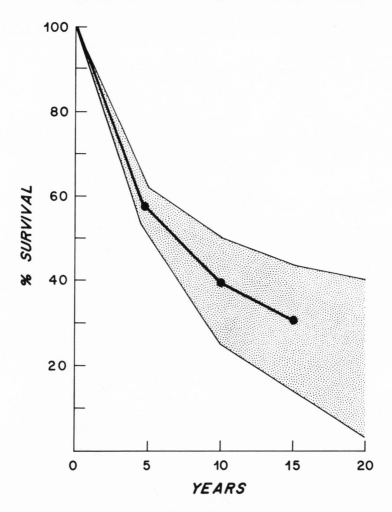

Fig. 5: *Percent survival following simple mastectomy plus irradiation — 15-year follow-up. (Data not corrected for life expectancy.) The shaded area represents the survival curves following radical mastectomy depicted in detail in Fig. 4 (Bruce[38]).*

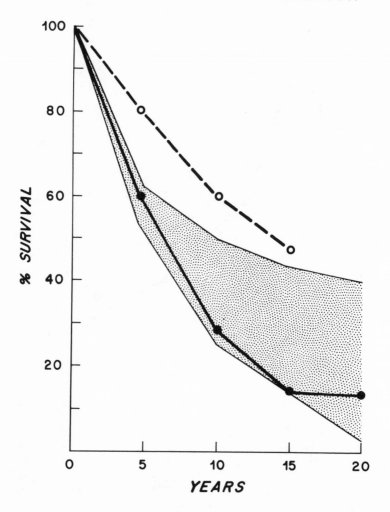

Fig. 6: *Percent survival after limited excision plus primary irradiation — 15-to-20-year follow-up. Broken line curve corrected for life expectancy (Mustakallio[39]). Solid line uncorrected (Peters[33]). The shaded area represents the survival curves following radical mastectomy depicted in detail in Fig. 4.*

tectomy suggests that this is the best that surgery can do. All of the operations of the six series, not just Dr. McLaughlin's, were carried out by expert surgeons who took advantage of all the modern refinements. It is inconceivable that another surgeon will come along at this juncture with a new surgical wrinkle to better the outcome materially. Surgery has been doing what it can, helping but not curing enough women. Surgery has shot its bolt. If there is to be improvement in care, it is not going to be by further surgery.

I am not saying that surgery per se is no good. I am saying it is not the method to be used as the principal treatment for breast cancer. Surgery is failing because the majority of patients have forms of the disease that do not lend themselves to surgical care.

One alternative to radical mastectomy, the McWhirter technique, introduced in World War II in Scotland, is half surgery, half radiation.[18,38] The surgeon excises just the breast without taking muscles or nodes, and the nodes are irradiated (see second section of Table 3 and Figure 5). A second alternative, also introduced at the start of World War II, by S. Mustakallio in Finland, is based on the local excision of the cancerous tumor, and treatment of the remaining breast as well as of the lymph nodes by heavy irradiation.[39] This places equal dependence on the radiation and the surgical removal (third section of Table 3 and Figure 6).[33-38] The results of both alternatives are identical with those following radical mastectomy — no better, no worse, as far as life expectancy is concerned.*

As the results of radical mastectomy are compared with those of the two alternatives, it becomes evident that any one of the three methods rids the breast and breast region of the cancerous cells and that their failure to achieve a better ultimate result must lie not in the therapies, but in the nature of the disease. The cancerous cells must have spread to distant parts of the body before the treatment, whether surgery or irradiation. The treatment came too late.

We can now see what is wrong with the so-called five-year

*In Chapter 7 I shall deal in greater detail with the above two alternative therapies, which depend to the greater extent upon radiation.

cure rate, the five-year point that doctors talk about and that patients are expected to take comfort from. It is commonly said that if the patient is well five years after the radical mastectomy, it is good news for the future. Just a glance at the mortality curves, following radical mastectomy, depicted in Figure 4 shows how shallow is the meaning of survival at five years after operation. By five years, 20 percent of the patients have already died, nearly as many more will have succumbed by the tenth year, and again nearly as many by the fifteenth. Even at fifteen years the end has not been reached; a few more patients will die before the twentieth year is reached. At best, but a third of the patients alive at five years will survive after the fifteenth year. To any woman who knows the continuing mortality of the disease, being alive and well at five years after surgery is small comfort, unless indeed her doctors know that her tumor was one of the least malignant (Type I), or unless the doctors have been treating her with antitumor drugs from the outset.

Present evidence indicates that the antitumor drugs are now changing this dismal picture, and what has until now been a five-year myth may ultimately become a reality. We shall deal more with this matter in the chapters on hormones, drugs, and immunotherapy.

In this consideration of surgery I have thus far not dealt with the disadvantages to the patient of all the radical procedures; namely, the damage to the motion of the arm and shoulder, the edema (swelling) of the arm, and the disfigurement and mutilation from loss of the breast. The loss of the pectoral muscles interferes with the motion of the arm and shoulder. The edema of the arm, no matter how slight, is all too obvious to the patient. I need not even mention the lymphangiosarcoma, a disastrous tumor that sometimes develops in the chronically swollen arm following a radical mastectomy. These physical defects are not to be minimized, nor are their psychological concomitants. Now that alternatives are available, all of these drawbacks, the physical and the psychological, must be taken into account by the doctors and patient in deciding on the therapy.

Since the results of surgical mastectomy, whether radical,

modified, or total, are no better than the alternatives, which lead to less disability and less disfigurement, the surgical removal of the whole breast in any form has no valid professional therapeutic excuse and is doomed, as the alternative methods become generally available.

The failure of both radical surgery and the two alternatives using radiation to achieve an acceptable relief of the disease emphasizes, indeed presses, the need to shift our emphasis from the local disease in the breast and regional lymph nodes to the disseminated widespread disease. Any one of the three methods, radical surgery or the two alternatives, is able to eliminate cancer from the breast and from the regional lymph nodes, but the widespread cells remain. The ultimate picture has, fortunately, been made altogether different by the discovery of anticancer drugs, and further comfort comes from the prospect of immunotherapy.

Chapter 7

Radiation

FIFTY YEARS after surgery, irradiation appeared as the first alternative therapy to surgery in the treatment of breast cancer and, indeed, cancers in general. Faltering at first, powerful, and sometimes harmful, radiation as a therapy received a bad name. However, with increasing knowledge and the adoption of more modern techniques, radiation treatment developed by leaps and bounds. In the last twenty years it has become the equivalent of surgery in the destruction of tumors.

For a long time the destruction of the normal neighboring tissues has remained a problem. But with the most recent understanding regarding the potential of high energy x-rays and radioactive particles whose radiation effects can be limited strictly to the tumor, even more is to be expected from radiation therapy in the future.

Soon after Wilhelm Roentgen discovered the x-ray in 1895, the destructive power of the rays was recognized.[1] Physicists interested in studying the nature of the rays, and doctors avidly seeking to use them as new diagnostic and therapeutic tools, soon found that their own bodies were burned by the rays. Everywhere in Europe and in the United States physicists and physicians who had engaged in x-ray studies developed burned hands and scarred faces.

The gradual harnessing of x-rays and of radioactive salts, such as radium and uranium, has a long and intricate history in medicine. Quite by chance I found myself in the front row in Boston when experimental physicists were developing instruments of possible use in the treatment of cancer. I came to know some of the ablest of these men, and at times I cared for one or two of them professionally. Two of my boyhood friends in Philadelphia were sons of William Duane, professor of physics at the University of Pennsylvania. In 1914 he was invited by Harvard to take charge of the research in the use of x-ray as a therapy for cancer. My contact with the family was renewed when I went to Harvard in 1920 as a student and roomed with one of the young Duanes. Then, as a medical student, in 1926 I spent a short time with Professor Duane in Germany, where he was visiting German physicists. Thus I learned at first hand of his achievement in improving the penetration of the x-ray while decreasing damage to the skin by raising the power of the machine from 1000 to 100,000 volts.[2] He understood the probable benefit of this increase in power but modestly left to others the description of what the machine could do. His work set the stage for the next act, when Robert Van de Graaff and John Trump of the Massachusetts Institute of Technology raised the voltage and the power still further, to one, then two, then three million volts.[3] As anticipated from Duane's observation, the one, two, and three million–volt machines allowed deeper penetration by the rays, and this permitted treatment of more deeply-lying cancers without significant damage to the skin. The first one million–volt machines were installed in 1937 and 1939 at the combined Huntington–Massachusetts General Hospital Tumor Clinic, with the first step up to 1.2 million volts in 1944.

Unfortunately, as has so often happened in the field of high energy physics, the technology outran the understanding of the dangers. When the 1.2 million–volt machine was set up, six members of the department of radiology came to see it in action. In the darkened room, the beam of charged particles was visible as it emerged from the tube. The radiation technician, a physicist, two of the residents, an interested staff member, and the chief of radiology stood six to eight feet away from the beam of light for less than two minutes. By nightfall it was realized that the parts of the men's bodies unprotected by clothing — face, scalp, and eyes — had all been burned. Not until this happened was it realized that the scattered beam of charged particles, cathode rays, were damaging to people, a fact later used to protect patients. I remember the event all too well, because I cared for the burns of the six men who had been in the room.[4]

Thus far I have concentrated on the search for new knowledge regarding radiation, and its uses in treatment of cancer that was taking place in Boston and Cambridge, at the Massachusetts General Hospital, Harvard, and the Massachusetts Institute of Technology. This was what I saw and learned as a student and young surgeon. All through my school, college, and medical school years important discoveries were being made in many parts of the world — Germany, France, Scandinavia, England, as well as Canada and the United States. I intend in no way to diminish by my account the contributions from all of these other countries and other medical centers in the United States.

Parallel with the development of the increasing power and penetration of the x-rays came knowledge regarding radioactive atoms, or isotopes. After the atom smasher, the cyclotron, was developed by Ernest Lawrence in Berkeley, California, a similar smasher was built at M.I.T., under the supervision of Professor Robley Evans.[5,6] As isotopes became available, medicine had new tools at its disposal. With the Manhattan Project and the development of the atomic bomb, the whole field of nuclear physics leaped forward. The development most important to medicine was the harnessing of radioactive cobalt, which was found to have a ray comparable in power of penetration with the two million–volt x-ray.[7] Since its cost was scarcely a tenth that of the huge, cumbersome x-ray machine, radioactive cobalt was purchased by hospitals and cancer centers the world over. Modern high energy radiation, therefore, became available to almost the entire population of the United States, wherever there were trained radiotherapists.

High voltage radiation was such an obviously useful tool that radiologists began to use it as a palliative treatment for breast cancer; that is, for cancers that had grown beyond the stage at which surgical removal could be accomplished. At the Massachusetts General Hospital, beginning in 1946, Drs. L. L. Robbins, M. Schulz, C. C. Wang, and their associates accepted more and more such patients. These women had large tumors with extensive metastases in their bones and liver. Irradiation was used to restrain and eliminate, if possible, the unsightly and painful ulcerating cancer in the breast. Frequently, at first, little could be done, but, as the radiation techniques improved, it became possible to eliminate the cancer from the breast entirely. The women were much more comfortable and felt much better about themselves for the time they had left.

Dr. Wang kept a careful eye on all of these women. By 1962, 97 had been irradiated and by 1967 a total of 221 had been treated.[8] In many cases the families authorized an autopsy when the patient died. Although the patient had usually died of the cancer's spread to other parts of the body, often the pathologists were unable to find any remnants of the cancer in the breast. The high voltage, high-powered x-ray, though unable to follow the cancer cells throughout the body, had wiped them out in their original site, the breast. This was an achievement not to be overlooked in the possible care of women whose cancer was not as far advanced as it had been in the 221 women first treated, and who wished to avoid the mutilation of a surgical mastectomy.

The radiotherapist today has many separate, distinct tools at his disposal.[9] Thirty years ago he was limited by low-powered x-rays and radium. Now, by selection of the suitable ray, he can direct the rays at small areas, even small spots near the surface or deeper within the body. He can limit the spread of the radiation to within half an inch or he can irradiate a larger body, such as the whole breast. At the same time he can spare the chest wall and the lungs beneath. He can also deliver exact, controlled doses, large or small.

These refinements are possible because he has at his beck and call beta rays, which penetrate tissues no farther than a centimeter, alpha rays, which are more destructive than the beta, and gamma rays, which penetrate deeply. Indeed, as many as 50 percent of the gamma rays of the two million–volt x-ray machine may pass on through the body, to be stopped only by a foot of concrete on the far side of the room. With such a selection at his disposal, the radiotherapist has only to choose what is suited to his purpose.*

In the use of a therapy as powerful as these modern x-rays and energy particles, one wonders why a dose powerful enough to destroy a cancer does not destroy the patient, too. In part, this is managed by the radiologist's care in hitting the tumor from several different directions so that little healthy tissue gets the full dose that hits the tumor. But in part, the radiotherapist is also making use of the special susceptibility of cancer cells. All cells are most susceptible to x-ray when they are in the final process of dividing, the so-called mitotic phase.[11] All growth in the body takes place by division of cells, and since a cancer is, by its nature, growing out of control, it is growing faster than the normal tissues around it, more cells are in the mitotic phase, and thus the cancer is more vulnerable than the normal cells to the radiation.

Normal cells, except in infants, when bodily growth is rapid, multiply slowly. There are exceptions, such as the lining cells of the upper intestine, but in adults most cells are static, as far as growth is concerned. They need to divide only to replace a worn-out, dying cell with a new one. A dividing cell is thus a rarity. In the normal breast, perhaps no more then 0.01 percent are preparing to divide at any one time, except during the growth period of adolescence or pregnancy. The normal breast tolerates, therefore, a moderate dose of x-ray.

The cells of a cancer, in contrast, are striving to multiply. Perhaps 5 percent are in the mitotic phase at any one time, and

*The list of rays and of energy derivatives has become a long one. In addition to the alpha, beta, and gamma rays of the x-ray machine, and special isotopes like radioactive cobalt, there are high energy particles, protons, neutrons, electrons, alpha particles, pions, mesons, and others still untried in medicine. These are produced by cyclotrons, linear accelerators, and synchrotons. The special qualities of these new sources of radiation energy have outstripped the capacity of the average physician to comprehend, and their use in cancer therapy has become a specialty within medicine's established specialty of radiotherapy. Those interested in knowing more may read an excellent review article written by Allen Hammond in *Science*.[10]

as that 5 percent are killed by the x-ray, another 5 percent have advanced to the mitotic phase and are then vulnerable to the succeeding doses of x-ray. The radiotherapist has learned to divide his doses and make use of this vulnerable period. He may divide his doses over five to eight weeks. The cancer melts away as dose after dose is given, while almost all of the normal cells survive.

There are other conditions of which the informed radiotherapist now knows to take advantage. One of these is the oxygen concentration within the tumor cells.[12] X-rays are most effective when the oxygen concentration is high. It is then that the cells are able to divide most rapidly. It is then that the number of cells in the mitotic phase are at the maximum and most vulnerable. As a tumor grows in size, the inner part of the tumor is farther and farther away from its oxygen source, the arterial blood. The oxygen level falls and the number of cells in mitosis declines. The larger the tumor, therefore, the less effective the x-rays against the center of the tumor. For this reason the radiotherapist, in treating a cancer within the breast, asks the surgeon to remove the mass or bulk of the tumor before he or she starts the radiation therapy.

We know that certain energy particles that kill cells by a different mechanism are apparently just as effective, perhaps even more so, when the oxygen concentration is low.[13] Useful in the treatment of other tumors, this knowledge has not as yet been applied to breast cancers.

Since x-rays are destructive, it should be clear that all cells, normal as well as tumorous in any phase, will be killed if a big enough dose is given. A dose exceeding the tolerance of the nondividing normal cells will damage the normal organ. The radiotherapist, of course, tries to avoid such overdose, but because the normal tissue of some human beings may be more sensitive than the average, some damage may ensue. For this reason, each patient throughout x-ray treatment must be carefully monitored.

In the endeavor to eliminate all cancer cells, it may be reasonable to destroy some of the immediately adjacent normal tissue.

Some damage to the normal skin may be accepted as the price for killing the cancer cells beneath. Obviously, the radiotherapist kills as little normal tissue as possible.

Since we have these new tools and new understanding of how and when they may be most effective, it should not be surprising that we are now able to destroy the cancer cells left in the breast after the primary tumor has been removed and also any cells in the immediately adjacent lymph nodes. That the effectiveness now equals the surgical removal of the breast and axillary lymph nodes should occasion no surprise. If eliminating the lymph nodes to which cancer has spread is truly important, as we have believed it to be, then irradiation has indeed an advantage over radical mastectomy, for it can also be used to treat the three other lymph node areas: the internal mammary, the supraclavicular, and the posterior chest nodes, which the surgeon cannot reach at all.[14,15]

Radiation has been employed in treating women with cancer of the breast in five separate ways.

1. From its advent x-ray has been tried in the hope that it will eradicate large cancers considered to have grown beyond surgical removal. Though the treatment may help, it also sometimes adds to the troubles. With improvement in techniques, Dr. C. C. Wang succeeded in eradicating some inoperable tumors within the breast, although he was able to do nothing comparable for the widespread disease.

2. For many years x-ray has tempered successfully the pain of metastatic cancer in bone.[16] At times it promotes the healing of a fracture at the site of a metastasis. Unfortunately, when a metastasis in bone is big enough to cause pain or a fracture, there are generally many such sites of cancerous spread that cannot be controlled by x-rays, and the disease marches on.

3. Irradiation is also being used as an adjunct to surgical mastectomy in its various forms. I alluded to the efforts of Keynes in London and McKittrick in Boston to improve the results of radical mastectomy by adding radium and x-ray therapy.[17,18] Their leads have been followed by many, and in the last twenty-five years it has been common in many circles in this country and

abroad to add x-rays, the so-called adjuvant x-ray treatment, in the postoperative weeks.

On present evidence such adjuvant irradiation appears to have done little.[19] It has not reduced the ultimate mortality or even delayed death. The reasons for its failure to contribute are now not hard to see. As far as it goes, surgery carries out its purpose of excising cancer. It should not surprise us, therefore, that when adjuvant x-ray is given following the surgical mastectomy, x-ray does not contribute significantly. Adjuvant x-ray in one sense is a kind of misfit, putting two therapies together when one alone is sufficient.

Adjuvant x-ray is given over the surgical wound, over the skin and the denuded chest wall. The dosage must be carefully limited; otherwise the operative wound will not heal. As we have seen, when a breast is removed surgically, the skin of the two sides of the breast is spared and is sewn over the defect on the chest wall. Such skin is divested for the most part of its blood supply, and must be delicately handled. It will eventually regain its blood supply from the chest wall beneath, but until then it is more vulnerable than normal skin to x-rays and drugs. The radiotherapist must therefore limit the dosage to half of the amount that he would usually give in attempting to kill all residual tumor cells. Similarly, drugs must be withheld for a time or the dosage reduced. Death of skin flaps has resulted from combinations of x-ray and chemotherapy.

In defense of the use of x-ray to supplement surgery, it should be pointed out that historically it was an inevitable step in the care of breast cancer. The adjuvant use was started before the full nature of the disease was understood; namely, that death was due not to local recurrence in the wound but to the distant spread of the disease. In the light of modern knowledge, it should be viewed as an anachronism.

4. Trying radium and x-ray as the sole treatment was perhaps the most important thing that Keynes did in the 1920s. He judged the results to be as good as those of radical surgery. His trials of radiation as the sole treatment were almost totally neglected. Although in themselves they did not lead far, they were

important because they laid the ground for the later, more extensive use of irradiation as the principal or so-called primary treatment.

With due credit to Keynes's initial effort in the 1920s, the pioneering use of irradiation as the primary treatment of early so-called operable breast cancer came first from Finland and France, then England and Canada. Almost no attention has been paid to it in the United States until very recent years. S. Mustakallio, a surgeon in Helsinki, reported in 1954 having treated 100 patients by removing only the cancerous tumor, a procedure known as lumpectomy, and following it by heavy irradiation of the remaining breast.[20] He started this treatment in 1940, on patients who had refused to accept the mutilation of a mastectomy. The results compared favorably with the course of 120 patients treated over the same period by radical mastectomy. For the same reasons, and also starting in 1940, F. Baclesse, in Paris, treated 100 patients, with comparable results, and in 1960 reported on his work.[21] In the meantime, in 1958, J. G. DeWinter of Brighton, England, had reported on a somewhat smaller series.[22] And from 1964 to 1974, several reports appeared, recounting successful use of this approach. Arthur Porritt, in 1964, and L. Wise and his collaborators, in 1971, reported from London.[23,24] M. Vera Peters, in 1969, described her work in Toronto.[25] Again, Mustakallio gave an account in 1972 of the fifteen-year follow-up of his 702 patients[26] (see Figure 6, page 72), and P. M. Rissanen, also of Helsinki, wrote up his research in 1973.[27]

In the United States, the surgical tradition has been so strong that most physicians and surgeons have been unwilling to yield the traditional mastectomy to primary radiation until the efficacy of irradiation is more evident. Ruth Guttman, of New York, has accepted for primary therapy those patients Cushman Haagenson felt would not do well with surgery.[28,29] Her results compare favorably with those to have been anticipated had the patients been operated on. Eleanor Montague, in Houston, has repeatedly advised the profession that irradiation is as effective as surgery and recently, in 1975, she reported her results with fifty-one patients.[30] L. R. Prosnitz and I. S. Goldenberg, of New Haven, have reported their experience with twenty-one patients, and E. Weber and S. Hellman with twenty-seven patients, both also in 1975.[31,32] Their experiences go back only eight years but they find the same thing: a survival rate equal to that following surgical mastectomy.

5. One more use of radiation remains, already mentioned in the previous chapter — half surgery and half radiation.[33,34] The breast is removed but muscles and lymph nodes are not resected. This is a simple mastectomy, now called "total." The lymph nodes of the axilla are then irradiated. The breast wound area may or may not be irradiated. This procedure was introduced by McWhirter, the radiotherapist in Edinburgh, as a war measure in 1940.[33] Many surgeons had been called to the army and few were left in Scotland competent to carry out the radical mastectomy. Sufficient physicians were available to manage the less demanding surgical procedure; radiologists and their equipment continued to be available. The results compared favorably with those obtained previously by radical mastectomy. After the war John Bruce carried out a comprehensive comparison of the two approaches with a fifteen-year follow-up.[34] His results, shown in Figure 5, page 71, were equal to those following radical mastectomy. Although this approach was at first disputed by many American surgeons, it is now generally accepted as an adequate measure. It has the obvious defect, like that of any operation removing the breast, of disfigurement and mutilation. It leaves the arm unscathed, however.

Now let us move to an account of the experience at the Massachusetts General Hospital with minimal surgery combined with primary irradiation to eliminate the residual local cancer.[35,36] The major portion of the breast is left intact, the only operation being the removal of the tumor and the tissue immediately surrounding it. The blood supply to the rest of the breast and to the skin over the breast remains intact. In removing the tumor, the surgeon is scrupulous in preserving this blood supply. Because of this precaution, the radiotherapist may with impunity give a full tumor dose to the breast and its environs.

At the meeting of the New England Surgical Society in 1967, two surgeons, two radiotherapists, and one pathologist of the staff of the Massachusetts General Hospital presented a paper on limited excision and primary irradiation as an alternative to radical mastectomy in the treatment of operable cancer of the breast.[35] Only twenty-seven patients had been treated in the nine-year period from 1956 to 1967, too few patients and too short a time to judge the efficacy of the therapy. The council of the society advised against publication.

From that time through 1975, the same team has increased its experience with limited excision to 180 patients, and the results were reported before the same society in September 1975.[36] In addition to the greater number of patients treated and more years in the follow-up, there were also developments in understanding, which changed the emphasis in the program of therapy. Foremost among these was the realization of the early widespread dissemination of cancer cells in the majority of patients currently being encountered in the United States.[37-40] The dissemination had apparently occurred before the patient was first seen, before any therapy had been carried out.[41] In view of this early spread, it was found that limited excision, followed by primary high energy irradiation, could be no better in saving life than surgical mastectomy in any of its forms.

Another development was that of antitumor drugs effective against many breast cancers.[42-45] The lethal properties of these drugs provide the first hope of cure, rather than of mere delay, in patients with early disseminated disease.

A third development has been the pathologist's growing appreciation of the biologic nature of the several breast cancers already described in Chapter 4.[46]

There are, therefore, four steps to our present program; those of surgery, pathology, radiotherapy, and chemotherapy.

Surgery. The first step is surgical; its six objectives and how they are to be met will be considered in detail in Chapter 13, on therapy.

The Pathologist's Study. At the close of the operation, the pathologist has the entire gross tumor, some surrounding breast tissue, and the lower axillary lymph nodes. He now needs time (three to four days) for a detailed study of the tumor and the nature of its spread. If the tumor proves to be noninvasive, the limited excision will suffice. The cancer of 10 of the 180 patients proved to be of this nature; they have received neither irradiation nor drug treatment. All are doing well.

If the cancer is invasive, the residual breast will need to be irradiated. Depending on the character of the invasion, the regional lymph nodes may also need irradiation. If the invasion indicates widespread dissemination, chemotherapy should follow the irradiation.

Radiation. The tumors of 170 of the patients revealed cells spreading out into the surrounding breast, some invading blood vessels, lymph vessels, or nerve sheaths. The residual breast of these 170 was therefore irradiated. Either because of lymph vessel invasion in the tumor, or cancer cells in one or more of the axillary nodes, the four regional lymph node areas in the majority of the 170 patients were irradiated — axillary, internal mammary, supraclavicular, and, when technically feasible, the posterior mediastinal nodes at the neck of the ribs.[14,15]

Chemotherapy. Since 1970 those women whose cancer was found by the pathologist to be consistent with disseminated disease have received prompt and prolonged chemotherapy. There have been thirty-five such women. How they were selected and how good their fortune has been will be considered in Chapter 9 on drug therapy. Most have done well, indicating that drugs do indeed provide a new hope.

There is no doubt in the minds of those who have shared in caring for our patients — surgeons, radiotherapists, pathologists, and medical oncologists — that limited surgical excision and primary high dosage irradiation offer, from the point of view of care of this cancer, an effective alternative to radical mastectomy or mastectomy in any of its forms. As far as the disfigurement or mutilation from loss of the breast, there is no comparison. Modern irradiation techniques are achieving a remarkable cosmetic result, and it is hard to imagine how a woman who has been provided with the evidence regarding the control of the cancer by the two approaches, surgical mastectomy and primary irradiation, and who has seen two women, one with the disfigurement of the total loss of a breast and the other with the partial loss and irradiation, could possibly select the surgical approach.

Complications. There are, understandably, limitations and disadvantages to radiation, just as there are to surgery. Both are destructive and both leave scars. The healing of a surgical wound is accomplished by proliferation of fibrous tissue that binds the wound together. Sometimes an excess of fibrous tissue is formed, resulting in a hypertrophied, or swollen, scar. Occasionally the fibrous tissue is so excessive that it is tumor-like and is known as a "keloid." Surgeons are careful, therefore, of how they make their incision and how they sew up the wound. If the incision can be run in the natural lines of the skin, the resulting scar is finer. If it has to be made at a right angle across the skin lines, the scar is thicker and more noticeable.

So, too, with irradiation. The scarring may be great or very little. Sometimes it is difficult for surgeon and radiotherapist to predict the amount of scarring. People's tissues react differently. The result of x-ray treatment in the breast of some women is scarcely noticeable. In others, there may be fibrosis within the breast, retracting the breast upward and more firmly against the chest wall. There may also be fine little capillary dilations in the skin, called "spiders" (telangiectases). Both the fibrosis and the capillary dilations are most likely to appear where there is an overlap of the fields of irradiation, where the dosage was doubled. The radiotherapist is at pains, therefore, to use the type of ray that is most effective and produces least scarring.

It is only fair to recall that the unsightly and unsuccessful results of the early use of x-ray in the treatment of breast cancer gave irradiation a bad name among physicians in the United States. Surgery, in contrast, was well performed, and the comparison of those early results led for many years to neglect of the potential of x-ray.

In our early experience in the 1950s and the first years of the 1960s, when the radiotherapist treated the breast with the tumor still in place, sometimes the surrounding breast was deeply scarred. What the radiotherapist can now achieve by the appropriate use of instruments and the minimally effective dosage is incomparably better.

The unsightly results of the earlier treatments were also, of course, discouraging to many women even though they retained their breasts. This discouragement was conveyed to other women facing possible irradiation. But this point of view has now changed. The excellent cosmetic results of modern radiation are bringing confidence to women and doctors alike.

The woman who is considering possible radiation therapy not only should be aware of the improved techniques but should also distinguish between primary radiation of the breast and radiation given to women in terminal phases of their disease or to cancers in deep-lying organs of the body, such as the liver or intestines. Radiation given as a last resort to sick, already debilitated women adds temporarily to their troubles. Primary radiation given to the breast does not reach the deep-lying organs and is therefore much better tolerated. Ordinarily, during treatment, the woman continues to consider herself well, stays at work, and is up and about, pursuing her normal activities, coming and going to the hospital for the treatments.

I am just old enough to have seen surgery at its height in the care of cancer by radical mastectomy. From my view, I have seen the confidence in surgery diminish and that in radiation rise. It would be foolhardy to suppose that x-ray or one of its equivalents will remain a principal therapy of breast cancer. Technique and complications aside, neither radical mastectomy nor primary radiation of the breast answers the problem of the widespread cells. For those distant cells, something else is needed. Drugs are proving so useful in demolishing cancer cells in general that even now one can see that much of our present use of irradiation may soon be supplanted, at least to some degree, by vaccination or other immunotherapy. As our understanding of what happens in a cancer cell increases, undoubtedly our treatment will change. Where we have used physical means, surgery or irradiation, we will increasingly be using drugs, immune measures, and perhaps more physiologic measures not even considered at present.

Chapter 8

Hormone Therapy

IN THE VERY YEAR of the discovery of the x-ray by Roentgen in Germany, the first attempt was made to treat breast cancer by removing the ovaries of two afflicted women. The surgeon was George Beatson; the place, Glasgow, Scotland; the year, 1895.[1] As a result of the operation the first patient, a woman of 33, enjoyed forty-six months of respite, only to have the cancer return to end her life.[2] The second patient, a woman of 40, failed to benefit, and died in six months. Thus was born the hormone therapy of breast cancer, antedating by a few years irradiation as an alternative or additional therapy to surgical removal of the breast.

Ever since 1895, the surgical removal of the ovaries has been tried again and again.[3-8] Sometimes successful in the premenopausal woman, the operation never helped after the menopause. We saw in Chapter 2 the astoundingly rapid subsidence of the cancerous metastases in the liver of the fourth patient, which followed immediately after the removal of her ovaries, and in contrast the lack of effect in the second patient; both patients were in the premenopausal period of life.

Beatson was not the first to recognize that the removal of the ovaries would diminish the size of benign tumors. Before Beatson's two operations on the patients with breast cancer, it had been well established that in women with fibroids of the uterus, removal of the ovaries resulted in atrophy of the fibroids. Surgeons caring for men had already borrowed on this experience with uterine fibroids by removing the testes of more than 200 men for the relief of the urinary obstruction caused by an enlarged prostate.[9,10] By 1903, resecting the testes had become a common operation, but it soon fell into disuse as operations on the prostate itself were perfected. In 1903, Hugh Young, of Baltimore, recorded removing the testes of two men with cancer of the prostate, but for this malignant condition the endocrine change brought no relief.[11]

Because of the unpredictable and temporary relief brought about by removal of the ovaries for cancer of the breast, the procedure saw little use during the first quarter of the twentieth century. This was the period when so much was expected of surgery. By 1930, when the limits of surgery began to be appreciated, efforts to find the possible role of hormones were renewed. New knowledge regarding the endocrine glands and their hormones was being reported from many laboratories, and for the next thirty years (1930–1960) there was an intensive search for a hormone cure of breast cancer. In addition to the two secretions of the ovary, several others, from the adrenal cortex and the anterior pituitary gland, were also found to influence the growth of breast cancer.

All these glands are internally secreting; that is, their hormones are carried directly to the places of action by the bloodstream. (They are variously called "ductless," "internally secreting," or "endocrine" glands.)

Of the many hormones, four are primarily responsible for breast growth and function: two from the ovary, estrogen and progesterone; two from the pituitary, growth hormone and prolactin. The adrenal cortex as one of its several functions secretes female hormone, providing a secondary source useful when the ovaries have been removed, or after the natural menopause. The woman's adrenal cortex also secretes male hormone, which presumably affects the breast in the opposite way much as the synthetic male hormone, androgen, is a known inhibitor of the estrogen action on the breast. There is evidence that after the menopause at least some of this male hormone is transformed into female estrogen, a further support to the woman.

The thyroid gland produces thyroxin, essential for all normal growth, particularly for normal breast development and lactation. The thyroid hormone is secreted in response to a special hormone from the anterior pituitary (thyroid-stimulating hormone, or TSH) and this pituitary hormone is closely allied to prolactin. Indeed, the TSH and prolactin overlap; both stimulate the breast.[12] This is believed to be the reason that breast cancer is found more frequently in patients with certain thyroid troubles, particularly an underactive thyroid, hypothyroidism.[13,14]

Also to be remembered is the oxytoxic hormone, which comes from a brain center; it starts the flow of milk, is believed to reduce the chance of ovulation, but has no known effect on growth of the breast cells.[15]

Then, lastly, there are those endocrine glands that do not directly or especially influence the breast but are nonetheless important to the well-being of women. These include the parathyroids producing parathyroid hormone; the medullary cells of the thyroid secreting calcitonen; the pancreas producing both insulin and glucagon; and the adrenal medulla producing epinephrin or adrenalin.

No account of glands and hormones would be complete without mentioning the recent discovery of a new set of chemicals, hormone-like in function but coming from brain centers and other tissues not traditionally endocrine glands. They are the prostaglandins.[16,17,18] Their life cycle is much shorter than that of most hormones, lasting only seconds to minutes. They govern such things as the stimulation of another brain center, or they put an end to the ovarian cycle if pregnancy does not take place.

Hormones and prostaglandins are messengers from their source to the target organ they are intended to stimulate. They chemically activate the target cells, and the stimulation continues as long as they are present.

In the last thirty-five years the chemical structure of almost all of these hormones has been determined, and this knowledge has permitted a widening understanding of just how they are secreted, what they do, and how they do it. The understanding, in turn, has resulted in many new strategies of hormone treatment for breast cancer, in the United States and also abroad.[19]

By 1920, it was obvious to physiologically minded physicians who were examining tumors that cancers were a miscarriage of the growth process and that a study of growth itself might well illuminate the basis and character of cancer. When David Edsall, the far-sighted dean of the Harvard Medical School, was looking in 1928 for a new chief to direct the research of Harvard's Huntington Cancer Laboratories, he elected to emphasize the growth process, and chose Dr. Joseph C. Aub. Dr. Aub had already distinguished himself as an endocrinologist, studying aspects of growth. In 1926 he was the first to identify the disease associated with excessive secretion of the parathyroid glands (hyperparathyroidism); and in 1927, with his colleagues, he described the metabolic effects on bone of overactivity of the anterior pituitary (acromegaly),[20,21,22] a disease marked by overgrowth of the bones and many other tissues.

The choice of Dr. Aub was of far-reaching consequence because he and his colleagues began measuring the endocrine aspects of normal and abnormal growth. In relation to breast cancer, for example, they studied the ovarian secretions of girls as they developed into adult women.[23] While they were doing this, the French chemist A. Lacassagne identified and synthesized the female sex hormone, estrogen.[24] Soon after this the male hormone, androgen, closely allied chemically to estrogen, was also isolated and synthesized. As soon as these two synthetic hormones were available, Aub and his colleagues assayed their effects on breast cancer.[25] The initial results were astounding.

In the mid-1930s a woman of 75 with many cancerous nodules extending from her breast out over the chest wall was given the female hormone; the nodules promptly dissolved, and normal-appearing skin healed over the ulcerations. But as Aub and his colleague Nathanson had anticipated, after a respite of nearly two years the cancer reappeared. They then shifted to the male hormone, which provided a second but shorter respite. Younger women with extensive cancer were treated with the male hormone; again, they gained unpredictable, at best temporary, relief. It thus became clear that some breast cancers were sensitive to female and male hormones given alternately.

These observations suggested that it was a change in hormone climate that induced the remission of the cancer. If a woman lived in a postmenopausal low estrogen state, then bringing her back into a highly female chemical environment was effective. The highly male environment induced by androgen, in contrast, was sometimes effective in the woman who was in her fertile phase of life or whose femaleness had been reactivated by estrogens.

Aub and others of his colleagues, W. D. Sohier and R. M. Kelley, now tried these same female and male hormones on cancers originating in other organs. But with the exception of cancer of the prostate, they were not found effective in any single instance. This was disappointing but not surprising because the tissues of the stomach and colon, thyroid and pancreas, are not subject to a comparable sex influence.

These classical observations of Aub and his co-workers were early in the understanding of the role of the endocrine gland in the treatment of cancer, and they were by no means the only studies that were going on. Lacassagne was able, by giving large doses of his artificial estrogen, to create tumors of the breast and uterus in experimental animals like the mouse and rat.[24] In addition to Lacassagne in France, there were many others.

Another outstanding advance came from Charles Huggins, in Chicago, in the 1940s. He was looking for a way to control prostatic cancer in men. He was aware, of course, of Young's trial, in 1903, of removing the testes. The presumed reduction in male hormone had not at that time appeared to help.

But Huggins was not to be put off. He was an endocrine genius, like Aub. He postulated that somewhere else in the body there must be another source of male hormone, a second line of defense for the man who might lose his testicles. Evidence in mice suggested that the source must lie in the inner layer of the adrenal cortex. If that was the case, it would be necessary, in order to eliminate all male hormone from a man, to remove the adrenal glands as well as the testes.[26]

The two adrenal glands lie just above the two kidneys. To remove both adrenals is hazardous, not only because of the difficulties of operation, but because two other layers of the adrenal cortex secrete hormones essential for normal life: cortisone, for the metabolism of sugar; and aldosterone, for control of the salts sodium and potassium. The operation was therefore a risky procedure until cortisone, the essential metabolic hormone for sugar, became available in synthetic form in 1952. With synthetic cortisone, Huggins was able to apply the operation more freely. He found it effective, as anticipated, in bringing about a resolution of both prostatic and breast cancers, but the relief was only temporary.[27] As with removal of the ovaries in patients with breast cancer, adrenalectomy helped only some of the patients, but cured none.

Following Huggins's precept, Nathanson, once synthetic cortisone had become available, applied adrenalectomy to patients with extensive metastases from breast cancer. The same layer of the adrenal cortex secreting male hormone also produces female hormone, and the removal of the adrenals in addition to the ovaries should remove all female hormone from the woman with the cancer. In some patients the initial results were dazzlingly successful. I remember these patients well; Dr. Nathanson was a close associate and I did the adrenalectomies for him. One patient, a 60-year-old librarian from Connecticut whose breast had been removed for cancer five years earlier, came to us in 1954 with her lungs filled with cancer almost to the exclusion of air. She began to breathe again as the tumor nodules shrank in the first days after the adrenalectomy. In six weeks the lumps in the lungs were no longer visible by x-ray and she returned to her job, saying she felt fully recovered. Nathanson and I were elated, but at the end of two years the cancer returned with a rush.

I should add that this patient was beyond the menopause. Otherwise we would probably have removed her ovaries before trying the more hazardous adrenalectomy. You will recall that in the fourth patient whose history was recounted in Chapter 2, we did remove the ovaries first with prompt and astounding effect for almost a year, and that with recurrence we then did the adrenalectomy. This second operation also helped, but much less and for a much shorter period. In contrast, the second of the patients described in that chapter received absolutely no benefit from either the ovariectomy or the adrenalectomy. Her disease progressed relentlessly. She went through both operations for naught.

In all, between 1952 and 1956, I removed the adrenal glands in eighteen patients who were suffering from extensive cancer of the breast. Six of them benefited strikingly, another six perhaps a little, and the third six not at all. During that same four-year period, Drs. Sohier and Kelley were trying further hormone manipulations, injecting cortisone as well as estrogens and androgens.[28] The benefits were the same as those following the adrenalectomy: one third of the patients improved; two-thirds did not. As a result, I stopped performing the operation after treating the eighteenth patient because the effect could be attained as well by injections.

Recently new drugs have been found that are better than cortisone alone in suppressing the adrenal glands. The combination of drugs and hormones makes the surgical operation even less necessary.[29,30,31] Besides, bilateral adrenalectomy is a horrifically big operation. It takes a lot out of the patient, who is already weakened by extensive cancer; and since its uncertain benefit is equaled by hormones and drugs, why perform it? Occasionally the operation is still recommended, but I judge it to be falling into disrepute. Too much for too little. We are not likely to hear of it much longer.

Having tried the removal of the primary sources of the sex hormones, in the ovaries and testes, and the second source, in the adrenals, doctors shifted the emphasis to the central governing gland, the anterior pituitary. It was reasoned that if the hormone climate was changed by knocking out the pituitary's function, useful life could be extended more than by any other endocrine maneuver, and perhaps even a cure achieved.

The anterior pituitary gland controls the majority of the internally secreting glands, and is itself controlled by the brain above it. It has been dubbed "the band master of the endocrine system." It is not as all-inclusive as that but its functions do affect the breast. It secretes the two hormones that stimulate the ovary (the gonadotropic and luteinizing hormones) and the adrenal stimulator (adrenal corticotrophic hormone). This last maintains the normal level of function of the adrenal cortex. Without these stimulators the function of ovaries and adrenals falls to a low level, almost as low as if all four organs — two ovaries and two adrenals — had been removed. In addition, the pituitary secretes all of the growth hormone and the prolactin needed by the breast for growth and lactation. Taking out the pituitary removes, therefore, all these breast stimulators in one swoop.

This operation (hypophysectomy) was championed principally by Bronson Ray, of Cornell, starting in 1954[32]* The effect of the operation lasts perhaps a little longer than that caused by the removal of ovaries and adrenals together. It benefits patients more than either ovariectomy or adrenalectomy but no more than half in all. It is another horrendous procedure, however, and the patient dwindles away into a precarious half-life, dependent upon daily administrations of cortisone, aldosterone, and thyroid.

Hypophysectomies, therefore, are also a big price for a short gain.[34] True, the gland centered in the skull beneath the brain no longer needs to be resected surgically. It can now be destroyed by accurately directed radiation. But this modern feat leaves the unfortunate patient in the same precarious life situation. Although it is still practiced occasionally as a last resort, removal or destruction of the pituitary may also be expected to disappear in the future.

To those who have watched a cancer of the breast shrink and disappear under endocrine therapy, seeing nodules dissolve and normal skin grow over in their place is nothing short of magical. No wonder physicians and clinical investigators have kept hoping that one day, if they could but find the right hormonal maneuver, breast carcinoma would be conquered and the pa-

---

*It is interesting to see how in medical research one thing grows out of another. Although removal of the pituitary was first reported by Rolf Luft and Herbert Olivecrona in 1953, it was Olaf H. Pearson and Rulon Rawson, two endocrinologists at the Memorial Hospital in New York, both of whom had trained with Aub in Boston, who pressed Bronson Ray to master the surgical problem.[33]

tient cured. Unfortunately, we know, based on reports from all over the world, that the cancers always have returned, most within a few years and all within fifteen.

The only reasonable explanation for this is that enough cancer cells survive to be the origin of the secondary growth. Either those surviving cells were insensitive to the hormone change, or they changed their metabolism sufficiently to survive in an insensitive form, and grow back.

Hormone therapy thus is not a cure, but nonetheless it has a great deal to offer to a woman already suffering from widespread disease uncontrolled by surgery, radiation, and antitumor drugs.[35] A respite that frees the patient of pain and allows her to lead a near normal life for one, two, or even three years is unquestionably a boon.

The hardship of the treatment falls on those whose tumors do not respond, or respond only for a short while. Recently, new methods have been found for identifying those cancers that will be sensitive, tumors with so-called estrogen and progesterone receptors.[36-39] The identifications are not absolute, but give promise for the future.

While we wait for further knowledge regarding the origins of cancer, for more effective antitumor drugs, and for possible immunizing vaccines, hormone therapy will remain helpful in the treatment of many women with advanced breast cancer. Increasingly, the hormone therapy of the future will depend upon identification of the tumors that are sensitive to endocrine change, on the ingestion or injection of several synthetic hormones, and less on operations like removal of the adrenals and the pituitary.

Looking back, it is difficult to see how so much could have been hoped for from endocrine therapy. Breast cancers are vicious, destructive tumors. Hormones, in contrast, are kindly, creative, and never by intent destructive. Indeed it is hard to see how an endocrine maneuver can on occasion induce even a temporary resolution. Perhaps the endocrine resolution is best likened to that which comes at the end of lactation, when thousands of gland cells are shed in the milk as the breast contracts to its resting state.

Chapter 9

Chemotherapy — The New Hope

THE COMING OF DRUGS has turned the tide in the care of patients with breast cancer from discouragement to new hope. In the preceding chapters we have seen that surgery has been unable to better its results in the last forty years. Capable of removing the cancer within the breast, surgery can do nothing about the cells that have become widespread throughout the body. Radiation, less mutilating than surgery, also can do no more than eliminate the cancer from the breast and breast region. Hormones, from which so much was hoped at first, have also failed to cure; they bring a respite only, and that to but one third of the patients. Now, drugs are the first effective treatment against those cells, lurking in bones, liver, and lungs, that ultimately kill the majority of the patients. Drugs are our first new hope in twenty-five years.

Antitumor drugs have been slow in coming to the fore in modern medicine, far slower than their counterparts that conquer bacteria, the so-called antibiotic drugs. The idea of drugs effective against both cancers and bacteria was conceived of at the same time and by the same person, the German chemist Paul Ehrlich, working in the years 1900 to 1910.[1] The antibacterial drugs emerged first, however, because the killing of bacteria proved to be a simpler problem. Bacteria are different from human cells, and it was possible quickly to find drugs toxic to them and at the same time in the same dosage less harmful to the human host. Cancer cells, in contrast, are human cells gone wrong. The cancer's aberration is little understood. It has therefore been harder to find drugs that will kill cancer cells and not at the same time destroy too many normal human cells.

German medicine was prepared for the concept and development of drugs against cancers and bacteria. The German pathologists in the nineteenth century described the intimate character of many cancers. After the discovery of bacteria by Pasteur in France, it was a German bacteriologist, Robert Koch, who identified the specifications that a newly discovered bacterium must meet to be termed the cause of an infectious disease. Ever since, these specifications have been known as Koch's postulates.[2,3] And it was the German chemists who led the way in the development of the world's chemical industry.

Ehrlich realized at the beginning that he could not test a drug on a sick human being. He had to have an experimental method. He and his associates spent the years from 1900 to 1906 in developing a number of malignant tumors that could be grown in experimental animals — rats, mice, and rabbits.[4] One of these, the ascites tumor of Ehrlich, is used to this day in testing. This experimentation was laborious, and Ehrlich's attention was soon taken up by the more productive work of fighting bacteria.

His work in this area flourished as he concentrated on the spirochete that caused syphilis. In the beginning, he knew that arsenic, mercury, and antimony were poisonous to the syphilis organism. He centered his research on arsenic, and made up one compound after another containing arsenic in various forms. Many that were toxic to the syphilis germ were also excessively so to the host, the human being. Finally, in 1909, after trying 605 arsenical compounds, he came upon arsphenamine, the 606th compound, lethal to the spirochete and comparatively well tolerated by the human being. This was an extraordinary find and "606" became the principal therapy for syphilis until the discovery, in 1943, of penicillin's greater usefulness.

Ehrlich did more than find the most effective drug against syphilis; he used a methodical empirical approach, testing one new chemical compound after another, and thus set the pace for the next major discovery of antibacterial drugs.

The German chemical dye industry from 1912 to 1918 determined to discover a drug that would be effective against the streptococcus, the bacterial scourge so prevalent in that period. Every single new chemical compound manufactured by the industry was tested for its ability to kill a streptococcus culture. Ten thousand new compounds were assayed before sulfanilamide was identified as the first effective drug against common wound infections.

Although sulfanilamide was first synthesized in 1908 by Paul Gelmo, an Austrian industrial chemist, its full significance as an antibacterial drug was not recognized until 1932.[5,6] In the years between, several related substances were produced by the German dye industry, many of them tested for their effect on bacteria. In 1932 it was evident to Gerhard Domagk, a dye chemist, that the sulfonamides were lethal, especially to the streptococcus, and the dye industry patented them under the name Prontosil. Appreciation of their value was slow. In 1935, Ernest Fourneau and his colleagues in Paris[7] reported the benefit of another sulfonamide derivative equal to that of Prontosil. But greatest credit is due to Leonard Colebrook,[8] of London, who in 1936 reported Prontosil's effectiveness against puerperal sepsis, the fever of childbirth. Shortly after, learning of Colebrook's success, Perrin Long,[9] of Johns Hopkins, introduced the sulfanilamide drugs to this country.

In this same thirty-year period, from Ehrlich's 606 in 1909 to the start of World War II, there was no comparable advance in antitumor drugs. The search for chemicals effective against tumors was being carried out in several laboratories, principally by A. Haddow, in the Imperial Cancer Institute in London.[10] Here he and his colleagues tried out cancer-causing chemicals to see if they could also kill cancers. They experimented as well with nitrogen mustard, a war gas from World War I. This work was set aside with the coming of World War II in favor of investigations dealing more directly with the war effort.

The next major advance in the drug field was the discovery of penicillin. While arsphenamine and the sulfonamides were found by the empirical method, penicillin, in contrast, was the result of a fortuitous observation of one man and the much later appreciation of that observation by another. In 1928, when Alexander Fleming, pathologist at St. Mary's Hospital in London, was growing cultures of staphylococci, one of the culture plates was contaminated by chance with the growth of a mold that inhibited the approach of the staphylococci. Fleming[11] described this observation and there it lay in the bacteriology literature until picked up in 1940 by Howard Florey, the professor of pathology at Oxford, who was looking for something as effective against the staphylococcus as the sulfonamides were against the streptococcus.[12] With the help of Ernst Chain, a refugee chemist from Nazi Germany, he was able to isolate the active substance in the penicillin mold. Not only did it kill the staphylococcus; it was as effective against the streptococcus as the sulfonamides and it was also much better tolerated by the human being. Under wartime urgency the chemical industry of England and the United States jumped in to produce penicillin in quantity. It proved to be a tremendous boon in the care of the war-wounded. Penicillin was the product of alert observation and the prepared mind; an approach, one might say, at a right angle to the empirical method used by the chemists in the discoveries of 606 and the sulfonamides.

The discovery by Fleming and Florey was immediately followed by search for other antibiotics growing in mold organisms. The cranberry bogs of New Jersey furnished tyrothricin and streptomycin, chemical substances effective against a host of separate disease-producing organisms;[13,14] and there are today more than two dozen similar antibiotics in use.

With the end of World War II, laboratories returned to the problems of tumors and the search for drugs effective against cancer.

Of course, penicillin and some of the antibacterial drugs were immediately tried. Penicillin was found to be erratically effective. Actinomycin, however, was early found potent against some tumors. Considerable attention was drawn again to the nitrogen mustards. During World War II, the solid chemical derivatives of the gas were discovered to be highly toxic and were conceived of as possible chemical warfare agents. They were studied in detail, therefore, and were proved to be especially lethal to lymphocytes and bone marrow cells. This selective action immediately called attention to their possible use in treating cancers of these cells, lymphomas and leukemias. Even though it was still wartime, investigation into their use was started, with the encouragement of the National Research Council. The preliminary findings were all encouraging.[15,16,17]

A host of problems needed investigation, and a collaborative program among cancer investigators was organized during the years 1948 to 1953, headed in an informal way by Dr. Cornelius P. Rhoads, director of the Sloan-Kettering Institute for Cancer Research of New York. But the ideas and ambitions of the laboratories outgrew the capability of private enterprise to carry them out, and with the development of the National Institutes of Health in Washington, the program came under the direction of the National Cancer Institute. Here, a huge collaborative program was developed to search for drugs effective against cancer.[18]

From 1953 to 1964, a total of 214,900 drugs was tested. Over the eleven years from 1955 to 1965, the cost of the federal cancer program, which included the drug-testing, came to a little over $1 billion.[19]

Every conceivable chemical compound was tested. The rules of testing were rigid: each compound had to be tried on at least three animal tumors and pass additional tests of possible toxicity before it was considered reasonable to try the compound on a human being. The program included investigators in England, continental Europe, and Japan, and this international collaboration has brought much to the program. The English, for example, have used a different set of tumor models from those of the National Cancer Institute and have been responsible for the discovery of the mycin drugs, actinomycin and, more recently, adriamycin.

In addition to the wide testing of all conceivable compounds, there have been, here and there, original ideas that have been especially profitable. A classic example of such an original discovery was that of aminopterin, a chemical antagonist to folic acid, which is a near relative of vitamin B12. Sidney Farber, pathologist at the Children's Hospital in Boston, had long been interested in cancer of the white blood cells, leukemia, in children.[20,21,22] In 1947 he was struck by the excessive number of marrow cells in leukemic children who had been fed folic acid in the hope of their being made better. In contrast, there was a paucity of cells in a child who before death had developed a folic acid deficiency. Farber immediately recognized the possible connection between folic acid and leukemia. Folic acid was making leukemia worse; its absence should improve it. In 1948, a chemist-friend, Subbarow, synthesized for Farber a substance antagonistic to folic acid, and this substance, aminopterin, proved, as had been hoped, a boon to children with leukemia. The white cells in their blood fell rapidly to normal with a prompt return of well-being lasting months and even years. Thus was born the group of drugs called "folic acid antagonists," which have helped patients not only with leukemia but also with many other cancers, including some with breast cancer.

So far, more than fifty drugs have been identified as being lethal to certain types of cancers. Some twenty of these are effective against one or more breast cancers; eight appear to be the most useful. It is anticipated that the separate types of breast cancers will be better treated by some drugs than by others. Much of this identification of specificity has still to be worked out.

A number of other discoveries made during the intensive drug program have turned out to be important to the breast cancer patient. Among these are drugs that inhibit the secretion of several of the hormones upon which the growth of some breast cancers depend. For example, Nafoxidine and Tamoxifin paralyze the action of estrogens.[23] Apparently they act by binding competitively with the estrogen receptor on the cancer cells and, by so doing, deprive the cells of the estrogen stimulation and support. Their effectiveness is limited to those patients who would have been helped by removal of the ovaries.

Similarly, a drug has been found that inhibits the chemical

synthesis of the adrenal cortical hormones, thereby making a surgical adrenalectomy unnecessary.[24] They thus give greater flexibility in the management of cancer patients, particularly those in whom the tumor has outgrown cell control by toxic drugs and who must rely upon hormone therapy.

There are also chemical ways of inhibiting secretions of prolactin by the pituitary.[25] These have proved not quite as effective as those that suppress the output of the ovary and the adrenal cortex, but still they provide an increasing number of measures useful in treating patients with more extensive cancer. Seemingly, our armamentarium is growing larger day by day, and is stocked with antihormone drugs as well as those that kill cancer cells directly.

Physicians frequently use the word "cure" in an ambiguous fashion in relation to cancer. When a surgeon has removed an acutely inflamed appendix, the wound has healed, and the patient feels well, the surgeon tells the patient that he or she is cured. Certainly with the appendix gone, there is no chance of another attack. So, too, may a physician speak of a patient's being cured of the common cold. Another attack may come some other day, but that will be a different cold.

Cure does not always have the same meaning in relation to a cancer. When a basal cell cancer of the skin is widely excised by a surgeon and he is sure that every cell has been cut out, that no cancer cells remain to recreate the tumor, he speaks of a cure. Another basal cell cancer may grow in another place, perhaps years later, but it will be a new tumor, not a return of the old one. In such an instance, cure is a reasonable term.

Not so with a cancer of the breast, which may hide away for years. Surgeons may speak of curing cancer of the breast when they have removed the entire breast and the axillary lymph nodes, hoping they "got it all." Or they may speak of a cure if no signs of the cancer have returned within the first five years after the operation (the "five-year cure rate"). And, indeed, for 25 percent of their patients, the operation really is a permanent cure. The other 75 percent still harbor the cells of the original cancer elsewhere in the body, and the disease eventually returns. The use of the word "cure" for this majority is downright misleading — misleading to physician as well as patient.

I have spoken of the new hope brought by the emergence of antitumor drugs. Just what does this mean? Does this mean cure or merely postponement of the eventually overwhelming growth?

Drugs against cancer of the breast were used first, of course, in those patients with whom everything else had failed. The disease was advanced; the metastases were extensive. The drugs judged successful caused the tumors to shrink, but none caused them to disappear completely — palliation but not cure. Yet, although but a last-ditch treatment, the drugs did prove lethal to cancer cells.

As the first drug trials were being carried out in human beings, experiments in animals revealed that the size of the tumor when treatment began had much to do with the ultimate success of the antitumor drug.[26] The smaller the tumor, the earlier the stages of its growth, the more successful was the drug in eliminating it. The type of experiment indicating the significance of size is illustrated as follows.

Eighty young female mice are inoculated with a set number of breast cancer cells that have been grown in culture. The mice are of a strain in which it has been proven that this type of cancer cell will grow, proliferate, and eventually kill the mice if the animals are untreated. To establish that the tumors are growing, at a stated interval after the tumor inoculation some of the animals, perhaps five, are sacrificed and autopsied. If all five show early but unmistakable growth of the tumor, the remainder are deemed ready for the start of the drug experiment. If there is any doubt regarding the success of the inoculation, there will be a further delay and autopsies of a few more animals before the drug experiment is started.

The remaining mice are divided into three groups of approximately twenty-five each. To the first group of twenty-five mice, a drug known to be toxic to this special type of breast tumor is given and the tumors are watched as they recede. At a set time

— for example, one month — a few animals are sacrificed and examined. If no tumor cells are found to have survived, the drug treatment is terminated. If there are still tumor cells, or doubt as to whether all have been killed, the drug is continued for another period — for example, three weeks longer — then is omitted. At stated intervals after the drug is stopped, an animal is sacrificed and autopsied to determine whether the tumor has in reality disappeared. When two or three such explorations have indicated that there is no surviving tumor, the remainder of the animals are allowed to live out their normal life span. As death occurs from usual causes, each animal is autopsied to see whether the cancer had truly disappeared. If no cancer is found in the animals of this first group after the drug therapy had been omitted, then this group is considered to have been cured of the cancer by the drug.

In the second group of twenty-five, the tumors are allowed to develop and grow to an unmistakable size, easily identifiable at sight. At this point the drug is started, the same drug and at the same dosage as given to the first group. The third group of twenty-five is set aside as a control; no drug is given to its members. Their tumors rapidly overwhelm them and they die. The tumors of the second group are at first diminished in size, but, after receding, begin to grow again despite continuation of the drug. The tumors grow, however, more slowly than in the control group, and eventually the mice are overwhelmed by the tumor, perhaps long after the untreated mice of the control group have died. The observations are: (1) that the tumor in the control (untreated) group is a lethal cancer; (2) that the drug delays the growth of the advanced tumor in the second group but does not eliminate it; and (3) that, in contrast, the early administration of the drug, when the tumor is still small — before it has reached the size of that in the second group — eliminates the tumor in the first group. The conclusions are that the drug, given late, only buys time. Given early, it cures the cancer.

Comparable experiments have been carried out in female mice of a strain prone to develop spontaneous breast cancer 80 to 90 percent of the time. Seventy-five of such female mice are divided into three groups of twenty-five each. At the first appearance of cancer-like lumps on the chest and abdominal walls, the lumps of six of the mice, two from each group, are biopsied, to make sure the lumps are cancerous. If they are, the first group is started immediately on the drug to be tested. When the tumors of the second group have grown to considerable size, the second group is then started on the drug. The tumors of the third group are allowed to grow free of interference, to determine the natural spontaneous course of the tumor. This is the control group; all of the mice in it die, overwhelmed by the tumors. If the mice of the first group survive, and autopsies at their natural deaths from other causes prove the absence of tumors, then it is reasonable to conclude that the drug had eradicated the tumors; that is, was curative. If the tumors of the second group regress when the drug is first started, but later grow again and eventually overwhelm the animals despite continuation of the drug, then the drug is partially effective but not curative.

There are two biochemical explanations for the greater success in smaller tumors: the concentrations of both oxygen and drug. A tumor derives its oxygen from blood vessels that enter the tumor from its periphery. As the tumor grows larger, the center of the tumor is farther and farther away from the source of oxygen, and as the oxygen decreases, the metabolic rate of that part of the tumor decreases with it. At the periphery of the tumor, where oxygen is abundant, the metabolic rate of the tumor cells continues to be normal.[27]

All cells, normal and cancerous, are especially vulnerable to drugs at the peak of metabolic activity, in the so-called S-phase, when the cell is doubling the amount of its genetic material, the DNA.[28] When living in low oxygen, the cell enters a metabolically inactive phase, and drugs are relatively ineffective.

In the discussion of radiation therapy, it was pointed out that cells were most sensitive to radiation in the mitotic phase, the last moment before a cell separates into two. Radiation has also proven less effective when the tumors are large; again, apparently, because the center of the tumor is low in oxygen and cell division is impeded. There are few if any mitotic figures. In relation to radiation therapy, therefore, it has been found best to remove the bulky tumors first; to get rid of the cells lacking oxygen. The same should also hold true in relation to drug treatment. So the surgical resection of the primary breast tumor before drug treatment is part of our comprehensive program.

In contrast to radiation, which is most effective only in the mitotic phase, an occasional drug has been found effective in the mitotic phase as well as in the S-phase. But this mitotic sensitivity has thus far been of less practical importance in the choice of drugs.

The greater sensitivity of cells to drugs during the S-phase governs the timing of the program of drug therapy in the way the mitotic phase governed the program of irradiation. Normal organs of the body are relatively insensitive, less easily damaged on any one day by drugs. Tumors, on the other hand, turning over more rapidly, have a greater proportion of cells in the S-phase and are, as a consequence, proportionately more sensitive to a drug administered on any one day. Also, since tumor cells are reduplicating continuously, on the next day there will be more cells in the S-phase to be knocked out. By repeated daily administration of drugs, as with daily administration of irradiation, tumor cells after tumor cells are killed as they mature to the S-phase. The normal tissues, in contrast, suffer little. The program of drugs thus covers many days, and many drug periods are advised. Patients who know this will understand why the drug treatment is designed to cover such long periods, with so many administrations.

The second reason why size is important is that the better blood circulation to the smaller tumors increases the concentration of the drug available to kill the tumor cells. In the center of the large tumor, not only is the oxygen diminished, but the concentration of the drug is also lessened.[29]

By 1970 our group at the Massachusetts General Hospital was satisfied that several of the anticancer drugs were truly effective in killing off breast cancer cells, and once we understood that the cancer was more vulnerable when it was small, we knew it was time to reconsider our whole program. For five years we had been using drugs as a last resort, but were not succeeding in eradicating the widespread cancer with drugs, probably because the metastic tumors were too large. To succeed, we reasoned that we must begin to treat when the metastases were tiny. But that meant that we must treat early, at the first phase of spread, before the cell masses grew large enough for us to see, feel, or detect by any known means.

We were also aware that three out of four patients had these lurking cells after their surgery and after radiation. We would have been justified in putting *every* patient on a drug program right away. But this would have meant that some people who didn't need the drugs would be getting them, even though by including everybody we would be saving more lives.

If by some means we could identify the one out of four who was already in the clear, already cured, she would avoid the trouble, risk, and expense of treatment. We suspected that the research and knowledge of our pathologists should be able to give us the means of making the distinction. At that moment, September 1970, a patient came to ask our adivce.

On September 17, 1970, Mrs. S.L. consulted me regarding a lump in her right breast, which she first noticed one week before. She was 55 years old, three years beyond the menopause. Her family physician had referred her to a surgeon who, she learned, would insist upon a radical mastectomy. But a friend recommended me, saying I would provide an alternative to mastectomy even if the lump proved to be malignant.

The lump measured not more than a centimeter and a half. The skin over it was dimpled and the lump was adherent to the breast around it, both signs of its being malignant. There were no enlarged glands palpable in the axilla and no palpable abnormalities in the opposite breast. X-ray mammograms indicated malignancy. X-rays of lungs and skeleton revealed no evidence of spread of cancer. The patient was frightened and overwhelmed. Before finding the lump, she said, she had been feeling well.

On September 22 I excised the lump with a 1-centimeter margin of surrounding normal-appearing breast tissue and the skin immediately over the tumor. A frozen section was done so that we could tell the patient and her husband the preliminary diagnosis. The pathologist reported invasive cancer. I then asked the pathologist to carry out the special stains needed to discern blood vessel invasion if present.

In closing the wound, I was able to leave the breast almost without distortion.

One week later the pathologist reported malignant cells invading many small veins within the tumor, positive evidence of blood vessel invasion. The tumor cells were of a medium degree of malignancy. There was neither a fibrous wall nor infiltration of lymphocytes at the edge of the tumor to suggest resistance to its advance into the surrounding breast.

Because the pathologist could see cancer cells making their way out into the normal breast, irradiation was decided on as the next step. Between October 1 and November 5, the radiotherapist gave Mrs. S.L. a full primary dose of irradiation, 6000 rads to the breast itself and 4500 rads to the adjacent lymph nodes.

While she was receiving the radiation therapy, a consultation regarding her future treatment was held by the representatives of the four different disciplines involved in breast cancer therapy. As surgeons, Dr. C. A. Wang, my associate of twenty years, and I reasoned that we had removed the mass of the tumor, and the only cancer cells left were clusters of cells farther out in the breast, perhaps in the regional lymph nodes and — if the pathologist agreed — perhaps widespread throughout the body. Then we heard the view of Dr. Benjamin Castleman, our long-time chief of pathology and one of the country's leading pathologists, and his younger associate, Dr. John Long. Because of the blood vessel invasion, they emphasized that cancer cells would have passed from the tumor in the breast directly into the bloodstream before the tumor had been excised and would therefore have been disseminated undetectably in various organs. Our inability to prove their existence by x-ray of the patient's lungs and bones did not mean that they were not there in minute clusters. I remind you that Dr. Robert Scully, Dr. Castleman's associate, had pointed out to me, in the case of the fourth patient described in Chapter 2, that the blood vessel invasion he could see in the primary tumor was almost certainly the reason the patient was found to have liver metastases eight months after the tumor and breast had been excised. That was back in 1963. But now, in 1970, our patient's tumor was as similar to that of the patient of Chapter 2 as such tumors ever are to one another.

It so happened that Dr. Long had had two years of his training with Dr. Lauren Ackerman, in St. Louis, where the importance of blood vessel invasion in breast cancer had been most clearly defined.[30] This special experience of Dr. Long has meant much, not only to Dr. Castleman, but to all of us in the breast cancer program.

The radiotherapist, Dr. C. C. Wang, was confident that he could eradicate the cancer cells left in the breast, but knew that if cells had already spread through the blood stream, he could do no more about them than we surgeons.

At this point, November 1970, the standard treatment of such a patient was to wait and see if metastases did indeed appear in bone or lung or liver, and then treat with drugs. Careful follow-up would be made to pick up any metastases at the earliest possible point. But now we realized that if we waited until we had this tangible proof of spread, the masses of tumor cells would be too large to be eliminated by drugs, the chance to cure the patient would have been missed, and the life of the patient jeopardized. If we waited, the best we could do would be a holding action, last-ditch treatment such as the endocrine maneuvers carried out in the patient of Chapter 2.

The chance to bring effective treatment was *now*, not later. We knew we would be criticized for departing from the traditional approach by treating something that we could not prove was there. Yet from our previous experience with patients whose tumors showed this same blood vessel invasion — and not only our experience, but that of Dr. Ackerman and others — we knew in all reasonableness that this patient must have such early spread.[31,32]

We also had to decide who could best carry the responsibility for treating Mrs. S.L. with these toxic drugs. Not the surgeon, not the pathologist, not the radiotherapist, but the medical oncologist, who is the expert — in this case, Dr. W. Davies Sohier. Dr. Sohier was, of course, at the center of the consultation regarding this patient's total program of treatment.

After completing his medical residency, Dr. Sohier had joined Dr. Aub in the cancer research laboratories in 1951. He became involved in the day-to-day care of patients with cancer, particularly in the management of drug therapy; and had been in the thick of the development and use of drugs since 1951, so he knew full well their value and limitations. His extensive experience had included treating women with advanced breast cancer, but neither he nor any of his colleagues up to this point had treated a patient with presumed but unproven residual cancer.

Together we reviewed with Dr. Long the pathology of the ninety patients treated by radiation without mastectomy between 1956 and 1970. Thirteen of those patients had had blood vessel invasion in the tumor; despite an otherwise good outlook for many of them, twelve had already died, and only one was alive in 1970. This finding was the worst omen of any we had encountered. It was in keeping with the long experience of both Drs. Ackerman and Castleman. Dr. Sohier was convinced; he saw the obligation and was ready to break with tradition.

On December 8 he started the drug therapy of Mrs. S.L. with injections of 5 fluorouracil, methotrexate and vincristine and cytoxan by mouth. For two and a half years Dr. Sohier continued the on-again, off-again drug treatment — three weeks of treatment, six weeks of rest. The therapy was completed in June 1973.

The patient accepted the treatment boldly. She even hesitated to go on a summer vacation in 1971 because she did not want to venture far from Dr. Sohier or interrupt the program of treatment. She was able throughout the two and a half years to function normally in caring for her husband and family.

The evening after the first injection she had felt nauseated, and the next morning she vomited. From then on nausea was not a problem, and at no time did she develop diarrhea or irritation of the lower bowel. Several weeks later, at the fifth injection, she reported occasional tingling of the fingers but no weakness, staggering, or joint pains. A week later, as treatment continued, she felt unsteady, as if "walking on air," but this feeling subsided at the next pause in treatment. She had only one upper respiratory infection during the two and one half years. She has been seen each six months since the treatments. With the exception of colds each winter she has remained well. At this writing, six and a half years after operation, there are no signs of further cancer.

The experience with the following patient, Mrs. D.B., illustrates what we had learned in two years of the types of cancer growth calling for early drug therapy. This patient also had a different set of reactions to the drugs used.

Mrs. D.B., aged 54, consulted me on December 12, 1972. Five days before, as she was standing in front of the mirror, she noticed a little fullness in her right breast, which she had not seen before. She talked of her breasts as quite small and thought she would have noticed any earlier change. She had not felt anything wrong, but she did not examine her breasts regularly. She considered herself perfectly healthy. She had seen her physician during the the summer and he had found nothing wrong with her breasts then.

Her periods had stopped some years before, she did not know exactly when; perhaps four to six years. She had not made note of it; she had had a very smooth, even time through the menopause. She was not, she told me, a person to give thought to her health other than to realize that she was healthy and always had been.

She was taller than average, thin, with high color in her face and clear skin. She looked well; her thyroid looked and felt normal. Her breasts were small but normal, with well-developed nipples. Her right breast felt a little fuller than the left, particularly just above the nipple in the middle. In that area three nodules could be felt, the largest just to the inside of the nipple line, the other two less definite. I suspected that the clearly palpable lump was a cancer, with spread to the other two lumps. There was a single enlarged lymph node in the axilla the size of a kidney bean, its size consistent with spread of cancer to it.

She said she was *not* anxious about the lumpiness, but whatever the lump was, she wanted to face the problem directly. Her behavior, however, gave her away; she was keyed up, answering my questions before I had finished posing them and asking her own questions quickly.

This was a woman with a physical handicap from birth. She had apparently learned early to make allowances for the disability so that she did not suffer from disabling embarrassment. Her prompt acceptance of the breast cancer suggested that the lifelong disfigurement had taught her how to deal with a tough, threatening physical problem.

She asked me straightforwardly what I thought it was. I talked with her about the meaning and the possible therapy. It was necessary to know, first of all, just what it was. I suggested that if the mammography confirmed my suspicions, the most direct way would be an excisional biopsy.

The Xeromammograms indicated a carcinoma and possible spread to the axillary lymph nodes. The left breast appeared normal. X-rays of the lung, heart, bones, and soft tissues were unremarkable. A bone scan with radioactive irridium showed no evidence of malignant cells in the bones.

On December 14, Dr. C. A. Wang removed the suspected lump above the right nipple. Gross examination showed it to be consistent with a cancerous tumor spreading out into the surrounding breast. The pathologist confirmed this on frozen section. Dr. Wang closed the short wound neatly in such a way that the defect left by the removal of the lump was hardly noticeable. Through a second short incision high up in the armpit he removed the enlarged gland. It, too, was consistent, on gross examination, with spread of the cancer. She returned home the following morning.

There was no doubt about the need to complete the treatment to the breast and breast region, either by surgical removal of the breast, or by irradiation of the breast and the lymph nodes that drained it. And there was no doubt in the patient's mind which she wanted. Starting early in January, she received thirty-eight x-ray treatments to the breast and lymph nodes. These were followed by irridium implants in March, which delivered an additional 2000 rads to the part of the breast where the tumor had been. In all, she received 6000 rads to the breast and 4500 rads to the lymph node areas.

What about possible distant spread and the need for drug therapy? There was no doubt about the spread of the cancer within the lymphatic system. But about blood vessel invasion, there was a difference of opinion. And even without blood vessel invasion, the lymphatic spread had long been recognized as threatening, and Dr. Sohier accepted her for treatment.

Since this decision in her case we have enlarged our policy to accept patients with lymph node invasion for drug therapy, whether or not blood vessel invasion was seen under the microscope. Three years later we have found that others in the National Breast Cancer Committee in the United States, and the Italian physicians in Milan, Italy, have undertaken comparable drug therapy with patients who have established lymph node spread.

Mrs. D.B.'s drug therapy was started by Dr. Sohier on January 3, 1973, and continued through three years on the intermittent off-and-on program. Three drugs were given by injection — 5 fluorouracil, vincristine, and methotrexate — and cytoxan by mouth. Later, the hormone prednisone was also given by mouth.

Throughout the first year of treatment the patient suffered intermittently from nausea, not enough to make her vomit but enough sometimes to make her choosy about the food she ate. The cytoxan was omitted by the tenth month, but this did not significantly alleviate the nausea. By April of the second year, the nausea increased with each injection, and the prednisone was added. This helped; so much so that she told us we should recommend it for all patients.

By October 1974, the twenty-first month of treatment, she felt well enough to go on a prolonged trip to the Far East with her husband. She took her drugs with her, and arrangements were made for her to receive the injections while she was away. She returned in February 1975, twenty-six months after starting treatment, feeling well, and ready to embark on the third year of treatment. This last she finished at the end of 1975.

Throughout the therapy both by irradiation and drugs she has continued without interruption the business enterprise she manages. She has maintained her home for husband and two grown children. At this writing, four and a half years after the start of treatment by removal of the tumor, she remains well, active, and without evidence of tumor.

There is no proof in these two patients, Mrs. S.L. and Mrs. D.B., that had we not given the drug therapy, they would have developed metastases. On the other hand, had they not been given the treatment, we firmly believe that they would have had recognizable metastatic cancer within two years. And, depending on the success or failure of palliative measures, they might well have died within five years. Whether we have cured the cancers or only stalled their growth we do not know, but benefited they almost certainly have been.

Thirty-five patients in all have been receiving drugs in this program since 1970. The results thus far have been gratifying but not perfect. Residual tumor has appeared in nine patients despite the drugs, and two of them have died. Clearly, the drugs used in these cases were ineffective. In the seven surviving patients, treated with changes of drugs, the tumors appear to be stationary. All of the others, twenty-six in number, continue well, without tumor, a remarkable achievement, considering the character of their cancers.

We shall need many more patients and many more years before we know the full usefulness of this drug treatment for women in the most threatened group.

We have learned more about how to choose the patient who should be advised to have the drug therapy. Our review of the cancers of patients who developed distant metastases that eventually overwhelmed them has helped us to establish a set of eleven conditions for instituting drug therapy. They are: (1) Delay in reporting. Any woman in the cancer age, over 35, delaying one or more months in reporting to a physician is at a disadvantage. This has long been recognized. (2) A tumor greater than 3 centimeters in diameter. The size means that it has been there for a considerable time. This also has long been recognized as disadvantageous to the patient. (3) Failure by the physician to remove the mass of the tumor in the effort to spare mutilating the breast. (4) Fixation of the tumor to the skin overlying it or to the chest wall. (5) Blood vessel invasion. (6) Lymph node invasion. (7) Lymphatic vessel invasion in the primary tumor even if the axillary nodes are negative. (8) Tumor invasion of nerve sheaths (perineural invasion). (9) A cancer of undifferentiated cells with many mitoses, indicating rapid growth. (10) Absence of a fibrous wall blocking the spread of the invading margin of the tumor. (11) No infiltration of lymphocytes at the invading margin. (These last two, numbers 10 and 11, will be dealt with at greater length later.) All eleven conditions point to a neglected or bad tumor, probably with widespread invasion controllable only by drugs.

We have built up our program of treatment step by step, slowly and carefully. First, the limited excision without mastectomy; second, the irradiation if the tumor is invading into the breast; and third, the latest phase, early use of drugs in those in whom distant spread is probable. In terms of experience in the United States, each one of these steps has been innovative; but it is supported by extensive experience in Canada and Europe.

Patients ask why we wait so long to give the drug; why we give the radiation first. It is unwise to give both radiation and drug therapy simultaneously. This has occasionally been done in the past and has resulted in excessive harm to the normal tissues. We have given the radiation first because it eliminates any residual cancer cells in the breast, which otherwise would be a continuing source for new distant metastases. In the future, it may be reasonable in some patients to omit the entire phase of radiation, but we are not certain enough about the effectiveness of drugs to make this move as yet. Our experience with radiation is longer, and we are confident of the ability of irradiation to destroy cancer cells.

Certain details of the program deserve emphasis. We have used multiple drugs, often in rotation. In this way, we believe, we are more likely to obviate drug tolerance by the cancer.

The drugs are given over a three-week period, followed by a

six-week rest. The rest enables the normal organs to recover from any damage they may have received. The recovery period allows women to stay at work and carry out home chores.

The patient is fully informed about the possible adverse reactions of each of the drugs used. Each drug is started on a low dosage and is increased until the patient notices an effect. This ensures that the patient is getting the largest dose she can tolerate. Tolerance for drugs varies from patient to patient; and it is important, since we are bent on killing the cancer, that we give the maximal dose, not a halfway dose that may not prove effective. As soon as a sign or a symptom is noticed, the drug dosage is either decreased to just below the symptom level or that drug is discontinued and another given in its place. In this manner, the woman is freed as much as possible of all symptoms.

The ability of the woman to fight off infections, such as the common cold, is also taken into account. Several of the anticancer drugs, for example, suppress the lymphocytes and white cells of the blood, important guardians against infections. This is called "immunosuppression," and recovery from it is a principal reason for the six-week vacation from each drug. Six weeks has proven time enough to allow the immune system to bounce back. None of our patients, fortunately, has had serious intercurrent infections, but the physician must be alert to all possible infections and to the need to add antibacterial therapy, such as penicillin. (This aspect of immunosuppression will be considered later in greater detail.)

Other forms of drug toxicity are also watched for. One or two of the drugs most used cause the hair to fall out, very distressing to any woman. Yet extensive loss of hair can be avoided by omitting the drug; or, if the patient is willing, the drug may be continued in lesser doses and the patient can wear a wig. In all the patients who have had any loss of hair, the hair has grown back promptly when the drug was omitted. *It is a short-lived, not a permanent, problem*. Similarly, a sore mouth or an upset stomach, muscle spasm or weakness, disappears promptly. So with all the complications. We have had no permanent symptoms, no symptoms surviving the omission of the drug by more than a few days. Hair loss is the one exception; although the hair starts to grow promptly, it takes a while to reach its usual fullness.

All of our present drugs — and probably those to come — are toxic. Their effectiveness depends on this toxicity. If they are given in too large quantities over too long a period, they will inevitably cause trouble. Such trouble is encountered in patients with extensive cancer when the doctor has pushed the drug to extreme dosages. In our program of early treatment when tumor masses presumably are small, we have felt we should avoid such high dosages. This means reducing the dosage or omitting the drug when the woman has symptoms, and, as stated, we also omit all drugs for a period to allow for recovery from the side effects. As long as the drug program is managed in this careful way, there is nothing to fear. You must be careful not to think of drug therapy as it may be used for some friend or acquaintance with advanced disease, for whom drug therapy is being forced as a last resort.

Our program has received gratifying confirmation from two large studies that employ early use of drugs: the National Cancer Institute's Breast Cancer Task Force under Dr. Bernard Fisher, of Pittsburgh, and the Italian group in Milan, under Dr. Bonadonna.[33,34] The drug treatment in all their patients was started immediately following radical or other mastectomy.

Fisher reported in 1975 a collaborative study, lasting eighteen months, with 196 patients, 99 of whom were treated with drugs, 105 with a placebo.[33] Bonadonna had 386 patients, 207 of whom received a multiple drug treatment and 179 of whom were untreated controls, included for purposes of comparison. All patients had previously had a mastectomy and four or more cancerous nodes had been found in the axilla. Fisher's placebo group did not fare as well as the treated. Bonadonna compared his treated group with the 179 patients who had had the mastectomy but no drugs. There were fewer recurrences and fewer deaths in the drug-treated patients over the three years of his observations.

One might well ask why the eight physicians at Massachusetts General Hospital did not ask to be included as one of the hospital groups in the collaborative research under Dr. Fisher's Task Force. In regard to the use of drugs, our courses are now running parallel, but the parallelism is only partial and recent. In 1966 we were invited to join as a collaborating hospital, but we declined, realizing that our philosophies regarding breast cancer were too divergent.[35,36] Fisher's study group was then, and still is, in favor of some form of mastectomy. All of its patients, like those of Bonadonna, have had either a radical or modified radical mastectomy before receiving the drugs.

By 1960 we believed we had seen the inadequacies and the disadvantages of total mastectomy in any of its forms. We could not in all conscience, therefore, join in the management of patients by a protocol of which we did not approve. We felt we should individualize each patient's needs and do as well as we could with each patient. In the long run, we believed, we would be more useful to our patients and to progress in the care of breast cancers as a whole.

A word about false hopes. The program to find effective drugs against cancer has been under tremendous pressure from the public and Congress.[37-40] People suffering from cancer, especially women with breast cancer, are all about us.

The pressure to produce has meant that an occasional drug has been released prematurely and on further evidence has had to be withdrawn. This recently happened to the drug hydrazine sulfate.[41]

Legitimate treatments develop slowly, and long-drawn-out suffering has led many patients in their discouragement to go to quacks — men and women with boxes supposed to contain miraculous instruments. In between such prematurely certified drugs as hydrazine sulfate and the quack boxes are occasional drugs or treatments labeled "scientific" by some and "quackery" by others. The stories of Krebiozen and Laetrile are such.

Laetrile, of which much was expected twenty years ago, has proven to be totally without effect on cancers and has become a notorious nostrum.[42] An extract of apricot pits, it has been used by an unscrupulous group to make great personal profit at the expense of the sufferers from cancer. It has held out false hope and has financially bled poor people for no return beyond the hope that something might come of it. Hardly an honorable way to take care of patients.

Dr. Robert C. Eyerly, chairman of the Committee on Unproven Methods of Cancer Management of the American Cancer Society, reported in January 1976 as follows:

Laetrile, identified as the chemical amygdalin and produced from ground, defatted apricot kernels and concentrates of apricot and peach pits, is not a new discovery. For more than 20 years, the proponents of this drug have claimed that Laetrile can "cure" cancer. For more than 20 years, these claims have been refuted by, to name only a few: the Cancer Commission of the California Medical Association, the California Cancer Advisory Council, the American Medical Association, the National Cancer Institute, and the American Cancer Society. The Food and Drug Administration has also reviewed the subject of Laetrile on several occasions . . .

In March 1963, the FDA reported that it had found "no competent, scientific evidence that Laetrile is effective for the treatment of cancer," and in 1965, the proponents agreed to a permanent court injunction against further distribution of the drug. A year later, the proponents pleaded guilty to violations of the injunction.

In April 1970, an Investigational New Drug Application to test Laetrile was awarded by the FDA, thus giving the proponents permission to obtain the drug for experimental and clinical studies. This was widely publicized and resulted in a resurgence of interest in Laetrile. However, the FDA review of the IND application disclosed a number of serious clinical problems and the IND was terminated in less than a month. Once again, in September 1971, an ad hoc committee of five oncology consultants independently reviewed and evaluated Laetrile and found "no acceptable evidence to justify clinical trials" of the drug. Shortly thereafter, the FDA prohibited the interstate shipment of Laetrile in the United States, until basic studies had been performed. The FDA *requested* that the proponents provide clinical records of patients treated with Laetrile. I believe four or five case histories were sent to the FDA, but they were completely unacceptable in terms of biopsy documentation and other scientific criteria.

Laetrile is still illegally available in the United States. In the spring of

1975, U.S. Customs officials uncovered an extensive international smuggling operation that imported contraband Laetrile into this country from Mexico and Germany.

Furthermore, in an attempt to circumvent the federal ban on Laetrile, the proponents have renamed it Bee-Seventeen, the "anti-neoplastic vitamin," and Aprikern. These oral preparations have been distributed to many health food stores across the country. However, the FDA has issued a public warning that they are misbranded and potentially dangerous; the ingestion of five capsules of Aprikern or two packets of Bee-Seventeen can be fatal in a child.

Despite such warnings, too many Americans have been or will be persuaded to use Laetrile through the propaganda of the proponents. To those of us who are deeply concerned with the welfare of cancer patients, the use of Laetrile rather than known, effective cancer treatments is the cruelest of all frauds.

Certain large underground agencies are extremely adept at promoting and publicizing Laetrile. They publish a journal, distribute leaflets, show films and hold conventions. Frankly, the promotion of Laetrile is an economically profitable business. In addition, the proponents have made it a "political" issue.

We, the "medical monopoly," the "cancer establishment," are purportedly involved in the "cover-up" and "suppression" of material. The proponents claim that we do not want to find a cure for cancer. In this time of public suspicion, such accusations are unfortunately given attention. It is difficult to respond to such an irrational statement. I can only reaffirm the American Cancer Society's commitment to the cure and control of cancer.

The scientific rationale is that amygdalin, split by the enzyme beta-glucosidase, releases glucose, benzaldehyde (a mild anesthetic), and cyanide, which is lethal to cells. Supposedly, cancer cells contain more enzyme than normal cells and thus receive a larger amount of cyanide. Normal cells are said to contain another enzyme, rhodanese, that detoxifies cyanide and therefore prevents unwanted destruction. However, there are many flaws in this hypothesis.

Studies have shown only traces of beta-glucosidase in animal tissues, and even less in experimental tumors. Furthermore, there is no pronounced difference in the level of rhodanese between normal and cancerous tissue.

Amygdalin administered parenterally [by injection] is probably excreted almost intact in the urine. Taken orally, it is decomposed in the intestinal tract by beta-glucosidase into highly lethal hydrogen cyanide.

Laetrile is 40 times more toxic when taken orally than parenterally.

Reports of Laetrile's ability to prevent, arrest, or cure cancer are, in the main, anecdotal. For instance, a prominent entertainer will claim that his wife was "miraculously" cured of cancer with Laetrile, while failing to mention that she was also treated with surgery, radiation therapy, and chemotherapy. For 20 years, we have asked the proponents of Laetrile for scientific documentation of efficacy, but it has not been forthcoming. Nonetheless, because of public pressure to begin clinical testing, Laetrile has recently undergone extensive experimental study by Sloan-Kettering Institute for Cancer Research and the Catholic Medical Center in New York, the National Cancer Institute in Bethesda, and Arthur D. Little, Inc., a research laboratory in Boston.

In 1973, Sloan-Kettering Institute conducted a preliminary experimental study which indicated that amygdalin had some inhibitory effect on the development of tumors and lung metastases in a strain of mice that develop spontaneous mammary cancer. Their findings were prematurely leaked to the press and received extensive publicity by the proponents of Laetrile. In an attempt to reproduce these initial results, two experiments were begun in 1974 at the Catholic Medical Center, using bioassay to verify data objectively. Researchers found no inhibition of primary tumor growth and no difference in the incidence of metastases between mice treated with amygdalin and controls.

Sloan-Kettering Institute has supported four additional studies of Laetrile. Two experiments attempted to entirely reproduce the conditions of the original study, even including the daily light cycle. Far from duplicating the initial findings, researchers discovered that the Laetrile-treated animals fared worse than the controls. Two later studies, which modified the original experiment, also had negative results.[43]

(The subject has also been covered in the June 7, 1976, issue of *Time* magazine.[44])

The current Laetrile experience is a reminder of the scandal regarding Krebiozen, a substance developed by two Yugoslavian brothers some twenty-seven years ago. The drug caught the attention of an older but, alas, gullible professor of medical science in Chicago.[45] Dr. Andrew Ivy was a medical scientist, not a clinical physician, and had not had experience with patients. He thought he saw miraculous properties in Krebiozen, but nobody since has been able to confirm them. There was a long bitter controversy, ending in a lawsuit. Unfortunately, Krebiozen just did not turn out the way it had been promised. It appears to have been a hoax.

It is altogether likely that next week another "miracle cure" will be reported, and we shall need to examine the evidence carefully, ready to accept what is substantial and good, but critical enough to discard those portions without foundation. Physicians must be open-minded and unprejudiced. On the other hand, the cancer problem is biologically complicated, and no jack-in-the-box treatment is likely to be successful.

Success in the search for antitumor drugs has brought new hope to patients with breast cancer. The search has been a long and biologically complicated one, more difficult than that for antibacterial drugs. Because the cancer cells are but aberrations of the woman's own body, it is more difficult to find a drug toxic to the cancer cells and not lethal to the woman herself. Viewed from this vantage point, the success that has already been achieved is extraordinary.

Present evidence indicates that the success of the drug program in treating widely dispersed cells will depend on introducing the drugs early, before clusters of cells have grown into larger tumor masses. We are also only at the beginning of our understanding of what makes a drug successful; new and better drugs will undoubtedly be forthcoming.

Side effects of the drugs have been bothersome but manageable. Patients have been able for the most part to stay at work or care for their households uninterruptedly. The comprehensive off-again, on-again program that we have initiated at the Massachusetts General Hospital is a two-year one, judged to offer the best hope for cure. If not cure, certainly a more prolonged restraint of the cancer's proliferation than has heretofore been achieved. Drugs do not necessarily displace the older treatments. They can be combined with hormone therapy and serve as an additional help to patients in the later phases of cancer treatment.

As with antibacterial therapy, the body's own immunity will undoubtedly prove important in the ultimate control of breast cancer.

Chapter 10

Immunotherapy — Immunity in the Prevention and Control of Breast Cancer

THE HUMAN BODY in its evolution has developed an extraordinary system of natural defenses. When attacked by an infection, a poison, an excessive exposure to the harmful rays of the sun, the body is able to muster a resistance to each. Attacks take many forms, and resistances are of many types.

In relation to the problems of breast cancer, there are two responses of obvious importance. The first is the development of an immune reaction to a cancer virus, comparable to the body's fight against the viruses of smallpox and measles. The second, of equal importance, is to cancers in which there is no viral element. The resistance is the body's capacity to destroy the cells of the cancer in a manner comparable to the body's rejection of an incompatible transplanted kidney.

Slowly, over the last few years, many scientists working in the field of cancer have come to believe that the identification of immune responses will be more important in the control of breast cancer than any other part of cancer research. There are some hard facts to bear this out, but it must be admitted that the belief is based a good deal on hope and a lot on conjecture.

The known, established forces of immunity within our bodies are complex and various. Not only do they ward off infectious intruders, principally viruses and bacteria, but they dispose also of abnormal cells and perform other duties not so well understood. All of these may be related in some way to the prevention and control of tumors.

As the possible forces of immunity against cancer are examined, those involved in the cause or start of cancer are of the most obvious importance. Few if any cancers have a simple cause. Involved are many factors, including sunlight, x-rays, chemicals, hormones, bacteria and viruses, heredity — and these are often in combinations, not one but several.

Sunlight is a known irritant that leads, after years of the body's exposure to it, to skin cancers in susceptible individuals.[1] Dark-haired people have the ability to form enough pigment to protect their skin. This pigment is, of course, that of suntan. The body has no known protection to x-ray, as it does to sunlight. The change in cell metabolism induced by x-ray may also lead later to cancer.[2] (Not everybody develops a cancer after exposure to x-ray and it is theoretically possible that in some individuals there is an immune process that prevents their getting into trouble.)

Chemicals also cause cancer by irritating cells, killing them in one way or another, and we know of no direct immune force leveled at eliminating the irritating effect of the chemical. We suspect, though, that there are immune forces leveled against the abnormal cell, created as a consequence of the irritation.[3]

The same is true of certain skin cancers associated with chronic bacterial infections. These cancers were not uncommon before the days of penicillin and other antibiotics that control the staphylococcus. The cancers occur in the skin around chronic sores.[4]

People who have long-standing ulceration in the intestinal tract associated with infection occasionally develop tumors at the site of the ulceration.[5] There is, however, no known carcinogenic stimulus resulting in breast cancer. For example, women who have had septic or infectious mastitis during the feeding of an infant do not have an increased incidence of cancer in the breast.[6] Bacterial infections are presumably not precursors of this disease.

Although hormones, particularly estrogens, are suspected of

playing a role in the development of breast cancer, there is at the present time no information regarding an immune response against the cell stimulation in the breast. Estrogens are, after all, secreted normally by the woman herself. Such a response is theoretically possible if the estrogen is an abnormal one, synthetic or from another animal and not quite like that secreted by the woman's own ovaries or adrenal glands.

Viruses have become a dominant theme in cancer research. This is due in no small measure to the discovery that a virus particle is responsible for spontaneous breast cancer in certain strains of mice.[7,8,9,10] The particle is transmitted through the mother's milk to the infant, who later also develops cancer.

A virus is called a particle, for it is not a complete cell organism like a bacterium, but a complicated protein molecule wrapped up in a membrane.[11] Alone, it is lifeless, and cannot divide and reproduce itself. To survive and multiply, it must attach itself to a living cell, plant or animal. Once attached, it invades the cell, multiplies, and takes over, breaking the cell apart; each new virus particle attaches itself to a neighboring cell, repeating the process until it kills the host or is stopped by an immune force.

A virus particle is too small to be seen by the ordinary light microscope. Bacteria, in contrast, are large enough to be seen, and bacteria are also visible in cultures, multiplying to form sizable colonies. Not so viruses, which live within the cells. Until the invention of the electron microscope, viruses could not be seen and identified.

There is no concrete evidence as yet of viruses in human breast cancer, although there are many reasons to suspect their involvement. If a virus were implicated with any certainty as a factor in human breast cancer, and the patient could be immunized against the virus, such immunization would be of great practical importance.

The most important use of immunity in control of a virus disease came in 1798, with the discovery by Edward Jenner, an English physician, of the relation of cowpox to smallpox.[12] Jenner observed that the milkmaids who contracted cowpox on their hands from milking cows did not later develop smallpox. He conceived of the idea of inoculating people with cowpox to prevent their contracting smallpox. Since then, smallpox has been virtually eradicated from the world by the use of the closely related virus of cowpox, which arouses the body's own immune reaction against smallpox.

Most recently, immunity has been achieved with certainty to other viral diseases — poliomyelitis, measles, and German measles,* each by a somewhat different method. But not to the common cold and influenza. In these acute diseases of the respiratory tract, many different strains of viruses are involved.[14] As many as sixty different strains of cold viruses have been identified, and several of influenza. Although a vaccine can be made against one strain, it is generally not effective against another. There is little or no overlap of the vaccines of colds or influenza comparable to that of cowpox over smallpox. So even if we are vaccinated against swine flu virus, we receive no protection if the epidemic is of the Hong Kong type. Unfortunately, it may well be that cancer viruses, if they do, indeed, exist in human breast cancer, will be of many types; and much work will be needed to identify the more frequent, the more virulent, and then find the specific vaccines to prevent them, or to stimulate their destruction if they have already obtained a foothold.

The human body has many additional and ingenious ways of holding bacterial and virus infections in check. Bacteria blown with dust into the eye are destroyed by an immune protein in the tears. Otherwise we should be plagued by almost continuous conjunctivitis. Similarly, the sweat of the skin of our hands kills off the streptococci; if it did not, we should have constant skin sores. So also the staphylococcus and colon bacillus are killed by the skin between buttocks and thighs. Were it not for stomach acid, which kills thousands of organisms growing in food, we would be poisoned far more often. The vagina is guarded by a bacterium, the Doederline bacillus, that helps kill off entering bacteria. Otherwise women would suffer repeated

---

* The immunities to these three have been the extraordinary gifts to humanity of Drs. John Enders, Albert Sabine, Jonas Salk, and their co-workers.[13]

infections of the vagina, uterus, and tubes, which might even lead to peritonitis.

The acute sore throat offers another example of the immunity mustered by the body. Most bad sore throats and tonsillitis are due to the hemolytic streptococcus, a ubiquitous bacterium. The bacteria are caught in the tonsils and other lymphoid follicles in the back of the throat and are promptly destroyed if the body is working well. The B-lymphocytes of the follicles make special immune proteins to attack the streptococci. If these fail, and the organisms manage to invade through the tonsillar membranes, the body's defense becomes more complicated. White blood corpuscles and T-killer lymphocytes collect to digest the organisms.[12] Fever is called on to accelerate the guarding reaction, and we take to our bed and use hot gargles to help the body fight the infection.

Immunity keeps many infections from breaking forth, including lobar pneumonia. This type of pneumonia is caused by the pneumococcus, another bacterium that, like the streptococcus and common cold virus, is transferred from one person to another by coughing or sneezing. Disappearing from our throat in the spring and summer, the pneumococcus is found in winter in the back of the nose, mouth, and larynx of 40 percent of people living in northern cities. Most of the time, the pneumococcus can do no harm because of the watchful guardians in our throats. But if we are chilled by falling through the ice while skating or being unduly exposed to snow and cold, our defenses are undermined, and pneumonia breaks out in a fulminating rush, with cough, sputum, chill, and fever.

Infections are not the only conditions in which the immune forces of the body are called into play. The common allergies to fish, strawberries, dust, cat hairs, and pollen are conceived of as overreactions to what were intended to be protective responses.

Such protective responses are probably not without meaning in patients with breast cancer. As is well known, patients with an allergy to fish develop a welt, or skin reaction, if an extract of fish is injected into the skin. Recently, the skin of thirteen women with breast cancer was injected with two separate extracts, one of a breast cancer and the other of the adjacent normal breast tissue.[15] Six developed sensitivity reaction to the cancer extract, none to the normal breast extract. From experimental evidence, we believe that such reactions will not be uncommon and that they indicate an effort on the part of the woman to destroy her cancer. How to make use of this response, how to enhance it, remains to be determined by further work.

Allergies are not the only noninfectious immune process that conceivably could be involved in patients with breast cancer. New evidence supports the belief that sometimes human beings develop an acute reaction to their own tissues under special conditions. Some physicians suspect that inflammation of the thyroid and forms of arthritis are such reactions.

The failure of this last type of immunity to protect the patient with breast cancer has perhaps been explained to some extent by recent experiments with cells of a human breast cancer grown in culture.[16] The patient had formed antibodies against the cancer, but when the antibody was extracted from the blood and added to a culture of the cancer cells, it failed to kill them. In a similar experiment with antibodies and bacteria, the bacteria would have been killed. The outer coating of these particular cancer cells, however, contained a sugar-protein combination, a glycoprotein, which apparently prevented the antibody from penetrating the coating. So the cancer cells lived on, unscathed.

There are, however, other evidences of immune responses in the human being with breast cancer. In the last decades of the nineteenth century and in the first half of the twentieth, many cancers were observed to regress spontaneously, and occasionally they were reported to have disappeared altogether.[17,18,19] Some few of the cancers were breast cancers of women. To the older physicians who saw and reported them, these experiences were enormously impressive.

From 1880 until 1950, the world medical literature recorded more than 400 patients with cancers that apparently regressed spontaneously.[20] The cancers were of all types, of the colon, the kidney, the lung, skin, and occasionally the breast. The sequence of events typical of the stories was that the patients, severely ill and suffering from the terminal phase of a cancer, caught an acute febrile infection, often caused by the streptococcus. Their fever rose; they seemed at death's door — when they passed through a crisis. Not only did the infection clear up rapidly, but from then on the cancer became smaller. Sometimes the cancer was reported to have disappeared completely; in other patients it regressed, only to grow again later. But to the observing physician there seemed little doubt that the acute infection had so stirred the immune process that the growth of the cancer was impeded.

Unfortunately, the descriptions of these experiences were not always complete. Oftentimes the diagnosis of cancer had been left in doubt for lack of microscopic proof, or the patient had been lost sight of and the ultimate outcome never described. In 1956, Warren Cole and his associate, T. C. Everson, reviewed 400 of these reports.[20] In only forty-seven did they feel sure that the patient had actually had a cancer and that, in fact, the cancer had really resolved or regressed. Too often the decrease in size of the tumor could have been due to subsidence of a peripheral wall of infectious inflammation, the kernel of cancer never having been affected. However, in the forty-seven abovementioned reports the claims of the describer were realistic.

Only four of the forty-seven patients had had breast cancer, and it was not clear, from the descriptions, that the cancer of these patients was actually cured. The cancer had merely regressed and then the patient was lost sight of; or if the patient died, no autopsy had been performed to see if the cancer had been eradicated. Cole and Everson suggested other possibilities that might have caused the regression, including an endocrine change. The ovaries or adrenal glands of the woman might have been destroyed by the cancer. We have encountered many a patient with breast cancer whose ovaries or adrenals were found at autopsy to have been destroyed by the cancer. Also, if the woman was in the premenopausal state, the coming of the natural menopause might have reversed the growth of the tumor. Cole and Everson felt that this might well have accounted for several of the reported regressions.

Cole and Everson's reservations are well taken, but nonetheless spontaneous regression, even disappearance, is an occasional happening, and points to the possible significance of immunity as a factor in control and relief of cancer.

A surgeon who had seen such spontaneous regression of tumors was Bradford Coley of New York.[17,18] Impressed by the preceding streptococcal infections, in 1895 he extracted the toxins from streptococci and other bacteria and began injecting them into patients with advanced cancer, hoping to gain relief for the patients. Sometimes it was judged that some relief was obtained. As a medical student and house surgeon, I was present at more than one visit Dr. Coley paid to the Massachusetts General Hospital, and I observed an occasional patient injected with his toxin. In that brief experience, I was not aware of any tumor that had regressed under the toxin's influence. It is fair to say that the toxin received a generous trial in several hospitals in the United States.

The pathologist looking through his microscope has identified cellular characteristics of some breast cancers that seem to indicate immune resistance on the part of the woman harboring the cancer. The principal evidence for such immune responses are cells of fibrous tissue, special infiltration of lymphocytes, and inflammatory-like changes within the lymph nodes draining the cancer.

The advancing margins of some breast cancers are surrounded by a dense wall of fibrous tissue.[21] The wall looks like an earthwork thrown up against the advance of the cells, holding up the spread of the tumor into the surrounding breast. It is a wall comparable to that seen surrounding many an abscess, such as a staphylococcal carbuncle, or the wall around a focus of tuberculosis. From these comparisons, the pathologists assume that the fibrous wall impedes the growth of the tumor.

Another anatomic sign believed by pathologists to indicate a reaction of the host against the cancer is an infiltration of lymphocytic cells at the margin of the tumor, just where the tumor cells are invading into the adjacent breast. The B-lymphocytes produce immune proteins, chemicals that kill unwelcome foreign cells. The T-type, called "killer lymphocytes," kill the cells and also act as scavengers of dying cells. The presence of both types suggests that they are fighting the advance of the tumor. In favor of this opinion, it has been noted that tumors with a pushing margin and lymphocytic infiltration at the advancing edge are generally more slow-growing than those in which the characteristics are absent. Hence, their presence suggests an outlook less dire than usual.

Swollen lymph nodes draining the cancer area, as in the axilla or under the breastbone, enlarged by an inflammatory-like reaction, are also believed by pathologists to represent an immune response of the host to the cancer and to be a good omen. The 36-year-old woman physician, the third patient described in Chapter 2, who had large lymph nodes that were mistaken for cancerous nodes, seems, in retrospect, almost certainly to have had such an immune response. A special cell called a "histiocyte" has sometimes been identified in such swollen nodes, and may play a part in such an immune response. In spite of the initial bad outlook, the young physician has done well, and it can be said that her body resisted and successfully repulsed the cancer.

For several years Dr. George Crile, Jr., of Cleveland, has warned against unnecessary, perhaps thoughtless, removal of the lymph nodes that drain the cancer area of the breast.[22,23] He feels that by removing the nodes or irradiating them, the surgeon may inadvertently be removing a safeguard. His experiments to test this point, reported several years ago, failed to convince the profession, and his theory was at first disregarded. But recently the Breast Cancer Task Force of the National Cancer Institute, under the two brothers Fisher, Edward the pathologist and Bernard the surgeon, has brought forward additional experimental evidence to indicate that lymph node resistance may be important in spontaneous breast cancer in mice.[24] The evidence is still too tenuous to be acceptable to many physicians. Perhaps our young physician patient is the most convincing proof that there is in some cases helpful resistance against the cancer from within the lymph nodes.

A number of experiments reported in the last fifteen years indicate that small animals, rats and mice, have the ability to develop an immune resistance to certain tumors. These include virus-induced mammary tumors. For example, a virus known to be capable of starting mammary tumors when inoculated into certain strains of newborn mice, but not in other strains, has been used to elucidate the difference in the metabolism of the two strains.[25] In the susceptible strain, inoculation with the virus is successful in starting tumors in 80 to 90 percent of the females. In the resistant strain, tumors are rarely induced in more than 10 percent of the females. If the thymus in the resistant strain is removed at birth, before the mice are inoculated, the inoculation is as successful, 80 to 90 percent of the females, as in the nonresistant strain. If later, when the tumor has developed, a thymus gland from another animal is engrafted into these thymectomized mice, the tumor may disappear completely. It has long been known that the thymus of the mouse in particular has the ability to produce a special type of lymphocyte, which prevents the successful take of the graft from another animal species. If the thymus has been removed at birth, the thymectomized animal is able to accept the grafted organ. This ability to resist a foreign graft is due to the presence of those special lymphocytes, the T-lymphocytes, so it is presumed that the failure of the graft in the resistant strain of mice with the thymus present is due to these special lymphocytes. It should be added that the effectiveness of grafting a thymus is limited, however, if the tumor mass has been allowed to grow too large. In other words, as in the use of drugs to eliminate experimental tumors, the mass of the tumor determines the success or failure of the immune process contained in the lymphocytes.

Several other experiments with virus-induced tumors indicate that the lymphocyte system is of particular importance in the defenses of the animal against tumor growth.[26] This includes not only the lymphocytes originating in the thymus gland beneath the breastbone, alluded to above, but also the well of lymphocytes in the spleen and the lymph nodes throughout the body.

The site chosen for a tumor inoculation is also important to the success of the animal in overcoming the growth of the tumor. Recently, George Prout, at the Massachusetts General Hospital, has succeeded in getting the cells of four human bladder cancers to grow in culture.[27] The success of the cells to grow and form a tumor in a rat inoculated with a given number of these cultured cells depends on the tissue of the site. If the cells are injected into the muscles of the leg, the tumor grows slowly, over a six-week period, to the size of a walnut shell, indicating clearly the success of the inoculation. If nothing further is done, the animal slowly overcomes the tumor; and in the succeeding several weeks the tumor totally disappears. If, however, the same number of cultured cells is injected into the peritoneal cavity of the rat — that is, the smooth, glistening space created by the peritoneum, which coats the intestines within the abdominal cavity — the inoculum grows rapidly, the cells spreading throughout the abdomen and eventually overwhelming the animal. The supposed immune forces ending the growth in the muscles apparently do not have sufficient time, or are not aroused by the tumor growth, in the abdominal cavity.

These observations lend credence to the pathologist's view that the lymphocytic infiltrate at the advancing margin of some breast cancers is, in all probability, an effort on the part of the woman's body to stem the growth of the tumor.

I have indicated the prominent place that viruses have acquired as probable factors in many cancers. Viruses have been clearly demonstrated to be the cause of several experimental cancers, most prominent among them the mouse tumor virus referred to above, which consistently initiates breast cancers in mice. The very number of viruses that have been identified as causing various experimental tumors has suggested that many viruses possess this property.

But more recent evidence has been gathered by David Baltimore, Howard Temin, and others, suggesting that the viruses that are truly causative of cancer in the human being are a limited group, having a special biologic quality, and that this special quality is shared by only a few viruses.[28,29] The large number of other noncancer-forming viruses are merely associated in the patient or experimental animal with the tumor, and are not causative. Baltimore and his associates have called this limited type of virus a "retrovirus"; he and others have found that the retrovirus has a special cancer-producing character enabling it to worm its way into a human cell and alter the DNA of that cell, transforming it from a normal cell into a cancer cell. The alteration in the DNA is difficult to identify in a human being but can be seen in the smaller less complicated mammals. Baltimore suggests this may explain why virus-induced breast cancer has been identified in mice but not in humans.

Efforts to identify viruses in human breast cancers having thus far failed, and with abundant experimental evidence indicating that certain tumors in animals do indeed incite an immune resistance, it is not surprising that there is a renewed interest in the possibility of immunizing women with breast cancer. The first program has been organized by the cancer centers of France, using BCG (Bacillus Calmette Guérin).[30] This material consists of live bacteria, in attenuated form, of the bacillus causing tuberculosis. It was produced by two French bacteriologists, Calmette and Guérin (hence the name), and has been widely used to immunize children against tuberculosis.[31]

Believing it beneficial in preventing tuberculosis, the province of Quebec has, for some years, ordered all children to be immunized with BCG. Review of the subsequent health of these children suggests that fewer have suffered from leukemia than children in other countries, not so immunized.[12] Taking a lead from this, the tumor group at UCLA has injected BCG into patients with malignant melanomas.[32] In many cases, in the short term, the melanomas have vanished. Others have reported similar success with melanomas and other skin cancers, particularly basal cell cancers.

At the present writing, the French physicians are trying injections of BCG in patients with breast cancer who have had a previous radical mastectomy, but the results are not yet in.[33]

Not long ago a group of experimenters in Houston tried BCG,

together with a three-drug therapy, against breast cancer.[34] A partial remission was observed in all patients, but it lasted longer in those in the group receiving the BCG. The report of the Houston study is a most hopeful one, confirming the thoughts and early experience of the French investigators. We may look forward to more extended use of BCG in the near future. It has not been tried, as far as we are aware, as a supplement in the early treatment of presumed widespread breast cancer.

In Chapter 9, on drug therapy, we pointed out the possible hazards of suppressing the body's ability to develop immunity; many of the drugs currently used in breast cancer therapy have that unfortunate side effect. Drugs kill rapidly multiplying cells most easily, and among normal cells the several lymphocytes and white blood cells are the hardest hit. Yet these are the very cells that contribute so much to the main defenses of the body against infection. Patients on drug therapy, as we have learned, must be particularly careful about possible bacterial and virus infections.

If some of the drugs we use against cancer also damage the body's immune system, which is in some degree restraining the growth of the cancer, why do we give these drugs? The answer is simple. The immune system as it is cannot hold the cancer in check, whereas the drugs work. Eventually it is to be hoped that we shall find a way to strengthen the body's own defenses so that the drugs will no longer be needed. The best we can do at present is the off-again, on-again therapy, which permits the immune defenses to recover and thus protect the body's other functions.

There are several important but little understood questions in the study of breast cancer that may be resolved as the field of immunity is further explored: the difference between the incidence of breast cancer in Caucasian women in the United States and Japanese women; the difference between the incidence of breast cancer in rural and urban women; and the influence of emotional stress on the incidence and course of breast cancer.

Cancer of the breast in women is five times as common in the United States as in Japan. Among the Japanese women who settled in Hawaii and California, the incidence has risen in each succeeding generation until, in the second American-born generation, the incidence is essentially that of the Caucasian population. The same low incidence is found in China; the same change with emigration to the United States. Every possible explanation for the discrepancy, including breast-feeding and diet, has been sought by epidemiologists. Careful analysis of others on both continents who have breast-fed has excluded this as a cause; the diets are different, but not sufficiently so to explain the different cancer incidence.

An aspect that has not been considered is the difference of immunity that people of the Orient inherently possess compared with those of the United States. People of the Orient have a high resistance to the kinds of infections that often appear as complications of surgical operations. They are able to withstand operations under conditions that in the United States would ordinarily be followed by serious wound infection. Their conditions of life, from birth on, may be the reason for this relatively high immunity against such common organisms as the streptococcus, the staphylococcus, and the colon bacillus. This high immunity of the Oriental may extend to the virus particles that may be the cause of many breast cancers.

In support of this conjecture about immunity is the fact that the women of Mexico also have a much lower incidence of breast cancer than those in North America. The people of Mexico have become inured to many infections, particularly the gastrointestinal infections that plague visitors from North America to Mexico. Immunity to these organisms has been found low or absent in North America, but obviously it is sufficient among the Mexican population to protect them.[35]

The incidence of breast cancer is less in rural women than in urban women in the United States, a difference noted in other countries as well. Rural residents, particularly those on farms, are exposed throughout life to more infection than those living in the cities. Minor cuts and bruises are less likely to become seriously infected in the farming population than among city dwellers. Could this immunity of rural people bear a relation to the lower incidence of breast cancer?

The incidence of malignant tumors is greatest in two phases of life, infancy and old age. Immunity is said to be lowest at these extremes of age. The infant is only beginning to build his or her own immune forces. Immunity dwindles as age advances, and is said[12] to be but 5 percent of what it was in middle age. Are these two factors related? They could be merely coincidental but nonetheless they are suggestive.

For many years emotional stress has been considered by some physicians to have a bearing on the incidence and character of malignant tumors, including cancer of the breast.[36] Dr. Edward L. Young, thoughtful senior surgeon of Boston in the first half of the twentieth century, told me repeatedly that the longer he lived in medicine, the more convinced he was that patients who were emotionally keyed up were more susceptible to cancer, and that those with cancer who were under especial emotional stress reacted poorly and the cancer proceeded more rapidly. In terms of immunity, both increased incidence and more rapid course of the cancer seem reasonable. We know full well that a person who is under emotional stress is more likely to succumb to the common infections. If a person is short of sleep from worry, he or she is much more likely to come down with the common cold. Pneumonia is also a complication of overwork and emotional stress.

Recently, the Pacific Northwest Research Foundation, in Seattle, found that mice exposed repeatedly to environmental stress are more prone to spontaneous mammary cancers than those allowed to rest quietly in their cages.[37] These experimental findings tend to confirm the long-ago clinical observations of Dr. Young.

By 1960, many cancer investigators were confident that a virus would be found to be a principal cause of breast cancer, and that if a vaccine could be produced against the virus, breast cancer in women would be brought under control. This confidence was based upon the unquestioned evidence that spontaneous breast cancer in mice was transferred from one mouse to another by a virus.

The search for a virus in human cancer has thus far failed, and investigators have turned back to seeking more knowledge about the fundamental biologic aspects of cancer growth. Viruses may exist but are obscured by the complicated patterns of malignant human cells.

Despite the negative evidence regarding viruses, there is much to indicate involvement of woman's immune system in the prevention and control of breast cancer. The evidence is largely indirect and of little practical use at present. But there are recent developments showing that substances such as Bacillus Calmette Guérin, which incite nonspecific immune responses when added to anticancer drugs, do effectively stall the growth of established breast cancers.

Such observations indicate that immune responses are important. Up to now, the responses are inadequate and not to be counted on for cure, since the patients ultimately succumb despite them. The observations are to be studied, however, with the hopeful prospect that effective immunotherapy ultimately will evolve. Until then, we are forced to treat as best we can.

Chapter 11

The Emotional Reactions to Cancer and the Mutilation of the Breast

CANCER OF THE BREAST is a special disease, a special disturbance, not just another cancer. It is a cancer with all the threat to life that cancer means, but it is far more. Treatment has brought such disfigurement that it is a threat to woman's image of herself.

The three patients of 1943 told me what their breasts meant to them. They adjusted to the loss as well as human beings can, but they taught me of the sacrifices.

In the years after 1943, I learned what mutilation means. As a physician I interviewed more than 200 women, each of whom had had a mastectomy, and to almost all, the loss of the breast has been tragic in some way. "Mutilation" is the exact word to describe what women feel has happened to them. By 1960, it was clear to me that there were two major problems facing the woman with cancer of the breast: the cancer itself and the mutilation of the treatment.

Over those same years, I watched the development of an alternative treatment, irradiation. It was used first to treat cancers that had grown beyond the reaches of surgery. In 1956 we tried it on the cancer of a woman who refused to have her breast removed, and it worked. We have used it again and again ever since. By 1960, I determined to do no further radical operations.

I have never known a woman who did not profoundly resent

the loss of her breast. The patients described in Chapter 2 are no exceptions. On the contrary, they are typical. The horror, the anger, the resentment, the depression, the bereavement, felt by the woman whose breast has been removed comes out sooner or later if the physician will sit quietly and listen. Some women are able to muster a brave front and say they are glad to be rid of their cancer. They say they have adjusted to the bereavement. But down underneath, the voices are not quiet.

The following is an example. As I was walking along the corridor of a hospital floor I noticed a woman standing in a doorway. As I came abreast of her, she moved to stand in front of me, blocking my way, and said, "Look at what they have done to me. You remember, Oliver, my breasts were small; but that makes no difference. They have robbed me of one." As she pulled her dressing gown aside to show the gauze bandage covering the wound of her chest where her breast and muscles had been, her words were loud and sharp and her eyes were fairly spitting fire. As I recovered from what was almost an attack, I realized that she was the wife of a medical school friend. The "they" she spoke of were her surgeon, a likable man, and her husband, a physician, who had permitted removal of the breast. She told me that a nurse had said I no longer approved of mastectomies. Three years later, when her young married daughter developed a lump, she insisted that the daughter come from New York to see me because she was fearful that someone might do a mastectomy. Fortunately, the lump proved to be a cyst. The mother's worry, of course, included the fear that her daughter might have inherited her cancer. Her worry, therefore, was not only concern over the possible mutilation.

There is no doubt that loss of a breast is a handicap to any woman. It is ridiculous to suppose otherwise. Every statement to the contrary flies in the face of what every thinking woman knows. The very idea of a mastectomy is devastating. The American Cancer Society's Reach to Recovery program is in itself an acknowledgment of this: recover from what — if not from the loss of the breast?

It is altogether reasonable that every woman should look with some resentment, if not horror, at the disfigurement. Women's breasts are part of her, the dominant visible part of her womanhood. They are comparable to a man's penis and scrotum, indicating that he is a man.

Every adolescent girl, as she grows up, measures her maturity by the development of her breasts. Breasts are something to be proud of or shy about. They are a part of her being as she emerges as a woman. Men physicians sometimes think that this is an overstatement, but I would remind them of themselves as boys at the swimming hole and how they prided themselves on their maturity. Those with well-developed penis and scrotum stepped forward to the diving board as if to say, "Watch me." And those less well-developed stayed in the background until fewer boys were noticing. Then, too, think how the adolescent boy beginning to shave allows his whiskers to grow a few days longer so that everyone will notice them. Girls have their own indications of developing maturity.

The breasts are not merely signs of physical and sexual maturity; they are part of woman's sense of herself as woman and mother. The young woman physician felt this sense of being. She had lost a part of her and this was the reason she demanded another child — to prove that she was still a woman.

Woman's breasts are part of her beauty. Every woman and every man knows this. It is not an invention of Madison Avenue advertising. It is nothing new. All we need to do is look at the beauty of Greek statues; the way the sculptor draped the woman's dress to expose a breast. So, too, with the art of the Renaissance, the low-neck dresses of the great painters, the hollow between the two breasts, the suggestion left by that hollow, sometimes one breast fully exposed, as in Titian's *Portrait of a Woman in a Fur*. It is not woman's idea alone that her breasts are part of her beauty. Man has told her this from the beginning of time.

Why wouldn't she feel bereft at the thought of losing a breast? If she has had the misfortune to have a mastectomy, why would she not mourn the loss of so important a part of her body? This is reasonable. The reaction has been so well expressed by a patient, 52 years of age, who had undergone a radical mastectomy. She wrote me:

Admirer always of the beautiful things in life — of the aesthetics, of landscapes, of shapes and colours, of works of art, I, myself, was and still am, after two years and two months, a hideous creature. It has been said that one gets over it, but with me it is a permanent, present, never-ending feeling. Curiously enough, the knowledge of having cancer didn't upset me — death is the only sure thing for us mortals — we all go one way or another. But for me life should be dignified and I feel diminished, disintegrating! . . .

To end this very long letter I just want to tell you, because you understand, that the trauma of mutilation is great. I am sure that some women take it better than others. Psychologically it has affected me very much; it may not show; friends tell me how wonderfully I have taken it. The joy of being alive has left me. I know I am a privileged woman in more than one way, but somehow I wonder if for the sake of living this operation should take place. I did it for my children, but now the once loving and understanding mother has turned into a nagging one, and certainly difficult to live with. They know it. I know it.

My work has been a blessing, for it has kept me overworked. Unlike other women who have only to think of themselves, I am lucky to have to run all day long.

For my daughter's sake, I sincerely hope that medicine will advance fast enough as well as for the millions around the world so that they don't have to go through this sad experience. Faith is important.

Woman's breasts are, of course, a part of her sexual feelings. Men also know this as well as women. Less significant to some, it is important to others, and not something that medicine can ignore as frivolous. It is there. It's a part of all of us and to be respected by medicine. The loss was especially difficult for a 45-year-old patient who wrote, five years after her mastectomy:

. . . The loss of my breast at such an early age has been a severe blow. I don't squabble with the Almighty's decisions, but if it had only happened 20 years later it would have been easier to bear. I have to be honest and admit it hasn't stopped me from doing anything I did before. I still ride, swim, work and take care of my home and husband. Even so, I always know it is with me, and this gives me some bad moments even now. My husband is and always has been my number one champion and supporter. He tells me that the fact I have only one breast makes no difference to him, that he is grateful to have me around, alive and well — and I believe him. But in our intimate moments, it is a hard thing for me to do to present him with this disfigurement. One breast by itself is rather obscene, I think. My husband says it doesn't look that way to him, but it looks that way to me.

I can truthfully say that the loss of a breast has not affected our lovemaking to any extent.

I've just realized that I have told a lie, but didn't recognize it until I saw it set down on paper. Our lovemaking so far as tenderness and wanting one another has not been affected, but my enjoyment of it has, because my left breast was always extremely sensitive and was one of my most important erogenous zones. Now it isn't there anymore, and I miss it to this day.

There is extensive American literature on woman's reaction to breast cancer and to mastectomy in particular. With few exceptions, the articles in the medical, nursing, and psychological literature deal with the problems of mastectomy, either the threat of it or the result of it.[1–25] An unawareness that was reasonable in the 1950s, before radiation had proven its value, is now inexcusable. This unawareness in the United States is due to a lack of understanding of the alternatives to mastectomy and what they would mean to the afflicted.[26–32] Those who for psychological reasons have recommended less mutilating operations, the avoidance of surgical removal of the breast in any one of its forms, can be counted on the fingers of one hand. It is astounding that women have not been more alert to the alternatives.

If one can accept that limited excision and irradiation are the equivalent of mastectomy in the care of the cancer, one can sweep away the great part of this dread of mutilation with one big swoop.

Not that irradiation is as yet a cosmetically perfect treatment; but it has come a long way. Compared with even ten years ago, it is much better controlled. After radiation, there are fewer dilated capillaries in the skin and less fibrous thickening in the breast; virtually none in most patients. In many, one can hardly tell which breast has been irradiated. And then this is to be emphasized: the results in the care of the cancer are just as good as those after any form of mastectomy. For the woman facing the problems of breast cancer, we are truly in a new era. It is high time that women and the physicians of the United States wake up. Why should women continue to suffer the dread of mastectomy? Why should physicians continue to impose this dread upon their patients?

It is hard to see why the surgeons of the United States have been so slow to examine the alternatives to removal of the breast. Why have American surgeons been so blind to the wound they leave, so thoughtless of the patient's feelings? In the first half of this century, when there was no alternative to mastectomy, the surgeon had to close his eyes and ears to what he was doing; but not so for the last twenty years. Over the past several years I have talked to many surgeons about woman's thoughts of her body and of mutilation. Almost all have argued with me, saying that I am too sentimental, and asking why do I make so much of it. To this question I have found an answer. I ask in return that if they had a cancer of the penis and there were two treatments, each equally good in the care of the cancer, one irradiation and the other surgical excision of the penis, which would they choose? They do not answer with words; they blanch out. The conversation has ended.

Thus, by turning to the less disfiguring alternative, we have gone a long way in answering woman's dread of the mutilation. It makes the whole problem of the cancer less fearful.

It is hard to overemphasize the importance of diminishing as much as possible the dread of the mutilation. It is the dread that keeps many women from reporting promptly to their doctor. If it is important for a woman with cancer to start her treatment early, and we know it is, then it is important that the medical profession respect woman's wishes about her body. If women know that doctors will try to avoid mutilation, they will report promptly, as they do for other cancers.

Some women will choose to have their cancer treated surgically by removal of the breast if their physician and surgeon advise it. They will feel that if the breast with the cancer in it is removed, then the cancer will surely be eliminated. But if they so choose, they should be aware that out of sight is not out of mind. The absence of the breast is a daily reminder that they have had breast cancer.

There may be other reasons for electing surgical mastectomy; a long distance to the nearest radiation facility, for one. Whatever the reason, the woman will be helped by learning beforehand of the possible emotional complications of removal of the breast.

When the radical mastectomy was the only treatment available, disfigurement was unavoidable and the ultimate outcome so disheartening that doctors found it hard to warn the patient of emotional complications of the operation and to discuss the course of the disease. The woman with breast cancer felt uninformed, and this often heightened her anxiety. But matters are now better; doctors may speak with optimism. The woman who has found a lump need not be driven into denial and neglect of herself.

With mutilation less of a factor, the cancer fears are still to be dealt with. Cancer arouses many worries, and many reactions to the worries. There is the initial shock and denial, resentment, anger, and inevitable depression. Then there are the obligations to the family, the unfinished tasks, the unfulfilled dreams and ambitions, the continuing uncertainty, and the concerns about impending pain and death. These are real, often harsh; difficult for the most stalwart to bear, particularly for the younger woman whose children, she knows, still need her. How is she to be helped with these troubles?

The moment a woman finds a lump in her breast she is not just startled; she is shocked. No matter how well-prepared we are, the knowledge that we may have cancer hits hard. The woman who has been practicing self-examination should, in one sense, be prepared for the finding of a lump. Then, too, a member of the family, perhaps her mother or a sister, had a cancer, and she fears that she lies in a high-risk group. Yet when she finds a lump, it is a shock; no doubt about it. It is fear of what the cancer will mean. "Is it growing rapidly?" "Will I die soon?" Until the nature of the tumor has been established, how can one not worry?

The worries can be so intense that almost as soon as they have appeared they are dismissed, relegated to the back of the brain, hidden, denied. This happens to almost everybody. It may be hidden for only five minutes, but more likely for days and even weeks. What does the patient herself make of this denial, and will she ask the doctor about it? He will point out to her that presumably the shock was unbearable, and of course it was reasonable to bury it until such time as the intensity of the fear was passed and it could emerge more quietly, in manageable form. It should be stressed that this happens to almost all of us, man or woman; that it is natural and in a sense wholesome because it allows us to recover our balance and proceed to plan with our powers of reason intact. The patient with breast cancer will not have suffered from the short time lost in getting on with treatment. The denial may have been helpful, not harmful.

Once ready to face the presence of a lump, a woman will want to consult her physician. She will want to know about the nature of the lump and the treatment needed. She should ask for reassurance about mastectomy and minimal mutilation. She will understand that it is essential that the true nature of the lump be established, and that this will presumably require a biopsy — but not a mastectomy. She must assert her right to be fully informed and to enter into the decisions. She could ask for time if she feels she needs it. The biopsy does not have to be done this afternoon or tomorrow morning or even before the end of the week. Time to think of the alternatives, to talk with her husband, daughter, sister, her family and friends. Time provides a breather, helping to restore confidence. A week's delay will do no harm. And if she wants it done sooner, why not? Nobody in his or her right mind likes an operation, and a biopsy of a tumor is an emotionally loaded one. Biopsy can be done under local anesthesia if the woman chooses. This will enable her to talk with the surgeon. On the other hand, some surgeons find it easier to cut out a breast lump if the patient is asleep under a general anesthetic. But many women are more comfortable emotionally if they are able to talk with the surgeon, to know just what is going on. A compromise is possible. The patient can ask the surgeon to start with local anesthesia. If this is found to be difficult, then she can ask him to give Pentothal and gas oxygen, and go to sleep. It should not take long, but the patient can be sure before she falls asleep that the surgeon understands her demand that the breast is not to be removed no matter what he finds.

When the biopsy procedure has been completed, there will be that time of waiting, hard to bear, for the final answer. But this waiting period offers the chance to reconsider the choice of treatment, a mastectomy or radiation. At every turn the patient will know that there is no dire haste; that time and study are more important than being in a hurry. If she is given time, she will not feel that she has been railroaded into having a mastectomy.

Undoubtedly, along the way the patient will meet a doctor, a nurse, a social worker, or other well-meaning friend who will ask her why she is electing one treatment over the other. She will have been made well aware that mastectomy is the traditional treatment. She will ask herself whether she is sacrificing the care of her cancer if she avoids mastectomy. "Am I being too emotional and silly?"

Somebody is sure to criticize her for being too emotional. Many doctors and nurses find emotional problems difficult to deal with, and will urge her to "be sensible," to "stop being emotional." But what are we all if not emotional beings? She deserves reassurance that to be emotional is human, that it is more helpful to express emotions than to suppress them; and she deserves a reminder that the nicest qualities of human beings are emotions, with kindliness, thoughtfulness, and generosity as examples.

The waiting period ends with the pathologist's report.

The woman whose lump turns out on biopsy to be benign has up to this point gone through all the worries of having cancer. At this moment she has been relieved of her anxieties.

The woman whose tumor proves to be malignant is now face to face with the decision regarding the next step in treatment. If she elects irradiation, and I shall assume that she does, she puts aside the dread of the mutilation of mastectomy and is freer to deal with the worries about the cancer itself.

When the biopsy wound is well along in its healing, two to four weeks, it will be time to start x-ray treatment to the breast. As the x-ray treatments proceed over the next five to six weeks, other emotional reactions are to be expected.

The change from mastectomy to the less disfiguring program has altered a number of the reactions. Anger is an example. Immediately following mastectomy, anger is prominent; it is difficult for the patient and for those caring for her. With irradiation, anger is far less. Milder and less disrupting to the patient, it centers on the question, "How could this happen to me — what have I done to deserve breast cancer?" It appears in various forms — sometimes complaints that the technicians are not properly managing the radiation therapy, that the radiotherapist has not paid sufficient attention or is not available as he or she should be for questioning and reassurance. The anger gradually disappears, giving way to depression and to anxieties about the future.

Depression is still common and must be alleviated. The anxieties take many forms and may relate to all kinds of unfinished business, to mates, to family and children, to many responsibilities.

Of enormous value in caring for all the worries are the personal contacts available during the daily x-ray treatments that the patient must undergo for five to six weeks. As she comes to know the radiotherapy staff — doctors, technicians, and secretaries — she can voice her concerns and, in return, receive encouragement from these many different people. (In our group, we are blessed at the present moment with a technician who does more than her assigned task of drawing blood from the patients for examination of their progress. The patients tell me that she is magnificent in her greetings and leisurely, supportive way. She encourages them to talk while she goes through her duties. She has that ability to spot a sore point, a troubling issue; and she manages the right word of hope and encouragement. Even if the doctor does not see the patient at each treatment, his or her presence is felt in a well-ordered therapeutic staff.)

The same kind of psychologic support comes if the patient is one who should go on to drug therapy. It is part of the routine of Dr. Sohier and his colleagues that the doctor sees the patient once a week; indeed, when she is receiving injections, he supervises or himself gives the injection. This affords the patient that very time she needs to ask questions, to voice her complaints and worries.

In addition to interchange between patient and professional staff, the radiation and drug treatments offer support in the form of her participation. As she comes in day after day for irradiation and, later, each week for drug therapy, she does so of her own volition. It is her choice to be treated in this manner rather than by surgery. She is participating. The treatment is not thrust upon her; her breast not grabbed from her. In many women this sense of participation has resulted in their asking, "Are you sure you've given me enough? If you think I should have more, let's go ahead."

These six weeks of irradiation and the months of intermittent drug therapy are difficult periods. The treatments are daily reminders of the cancer. At no time is the patient really free of worry and the need for psychologic support.

It sometimes seems as if a person could not worry intensely about more than one thing at a time. The worries of a patient with breast cancer often follow a sequence that suggests a process of a new worry arising to overshadow an old.

A woman in her mid-50s was increasingly worried about repeated lumps she had noticed over several years in both breasts. An aunt had had a breast removed for cancer ten years before. Two years earlier, her older sister had developed a cancer, and despite a mastectomy had recently died of the cancer. The patient's breasts were large and many nodules could be felt. One in her right breast was of particular concern, and bilateral mammograms were taken. Old fibrous thickenings were seen but no sign of cancer. Eight months later she felt a new lump in her other breast. A repeat mammogram was taken, and there, sure enough, was a tiny shadow not picked up on the previous plates. I advised limited excision and irradiation; a surgeon in her home town advised a radical mastectomy. Perplexed, she consulted two further surgeons, both of whom advised the radical operation. Her brother and sister-in-law urged the operation. She was in more of a stew than ever, but finally decided that keeping her breast was more important. My long-time associate, Dr. C. A. Wang, did an excisional biopsy. The tumor proved to be invasive cancer. She received the irradiation to the breast, and subsequently the prolonged course of drug therapy. Her first intense worry was over losing her breast. With that question settled, she turned to worry over the cancer and whether the drugs would be sufficient treatment. In the middle of the drug therapy, her husband developed acute infection in his colon and intestinal obstruction. In her worry over him, she virtually forgot about her cancer. In one sense it is fortunate that she has had to continue to focus on him, his continuing troubles, and the care of his colostomy.

A similar change of focus has long been known to occur in relation to pain. If a person who has suffered throughout his or her life from severe migraine headaches develops a second severe pain, the migraine disappears. Once the second pain is relieved, the migraine generally recurs.

After the x-ray and drug treatments comes the long haul. How can we prepare for that? If we knew absolutely how each cancer was behaving, how each had responded to treatment, we would be on firm footing. But the cancers vary, and there are surprises.

Recent studies of the pathology fortunately give us much needed knowledge.[33-34] First, it can be predicted with assurance that certain cancers will have been eliminated, and second, that others, despite treatment, will be likely to reappear. The psychologic and social support needed by patients whose cancers are within either of these two groups obviously differs, but each is equally important. The woman who can count on cure should be helped to realize this, and not be allowed to continue in unnecessary fear. The woman whose cancer is likely to return must be forewarned, and assured that the other therapies, such as endocrine changes or different drugs, are being held in readiness, that all hope is not lost. Psychologic support for her is, of course, difficult to give. She does not have to hear everything bad all at once. The door should be left open for her to ask, when she feels ready to hear more. In this way she is encouraged to take part in the planning of her care. If the cancer does grow out of hand, she must be helped to realize that her physician is beside her to give her whatever drugs are needed to shield her from pain; that if she wishes, no extreme measures will be taken. She should be encouraged, given every opportunity to discuss whatever problem occurs to her, offered a Living Will if it seems that might be her choice.

For those women whose cancers lie between the first and second groups, between the extremes of cure and probable return, the sequence of anxieties calling for psychologic and social support is variable and not predictable. Most will do well. For all, one matter is outstanding — there is far more hope now than there would have been fifteen or even ten years ago. Painstaking, regular medical checkups are mandatory. In that minority in whom the cancer was not eradicated, at least the later therapies will be instituted at the earliest sign of regrowth, and a reprieve obtained.

The period of watchfulness for this middle group will be long. Social planning will be needed. Psychological or emotional care will be even more important. The planning and care can take several forms. Visits to professional counselors — social workers, psychiatrists, or understanding family practitioners — may be wise. The family, too, needs thought, and in many cases constant attention. A worried husband or child must be helped to find a doctor or other counselor he may call on the telephone or go to consult. The children particularly are to be thought of, for they have the future responsibility. If they are not already aware of this, they must be alerted to their mother's need of support and to their own futures. They must understand why the therapy is being given and they too should share in the hope that now comes with drugs and possible immunotherapy.

Friends are not to be excluded. Oftentimes a friend has a more objective grasp of the situation than a member of the family, and can help enormously by guiding the patient's attention to the priorities, helping her to dismiss anxieties about less important matters, above all helping her to talk about herself, her illness, her continuing obligations, and her impending death.

Over the last few years I have been much impressed with

what some patients have told me they have gained from meditation — transcendental meditation or other forms. I strongly recommend it.

I found a lump in my left breast in 1964, just as I was preparing for an extended trip with my husband. I explored the situation with several surgeons and in the end decided to have a lumpectomy and subsequent radiation treatment. It was clear to me, when offered a choice, that to preserve my breast, and so part of my physical sexual being, was a vital concern and worth the risk involved in rejecting the orthodox form of treatment. My confidence was firm. I was aware that statistically the chances of cure were about fifty-fifty either way. Who would then opt for mutilation?

The choice involved risk which I willingly accepted. The radiation treatments served to keep me emotionally connected both with the radiologist and the surgeon. I experienced also the support of the nurses and technicians, as well as a deep sense of sharing with the others there for treatment. This experience deepened my sense of being one of many human beings for whom this experience was illuminating . . . facing the truth of the brevity of life.

I had for several years been realizing that the later years of one's life should and could be of a different character than the earlier times. The model I found was that of the Hindu world, where there are four stages to human life. The first is childhood, the second young adulthood when one enters marriage or a career, the third when one carries out one's role in society, and the fourth when one has earned the right to turn one's thoughts to the deepening of the inner life and the preparation for death.

This model has not been familiar in the West but recently, as a result of work with the terminally ill, interest in the experience of dying has been growing. It is, however, not the dying but the living process that can invade these later years. The turning inward can take the form of meditation, of reflecting on the meaning of one's life, and a deepening joy in all that has been experienced, even though much of it may have been difficult and sad. There is something about the process of having gone through it and survived that brings its own sense of elation.

The onset of breast cancer, after the first shock, served as a springboard for me into a new way of living. It has been the greatest aid to growth. Now indeed the ideas I had been entertaining of living differently became urgent. The time might be short. None of it could be wasted. I began to rethink my priorities.

The first priority became the practice of daily meditation. Each morning I set aside a quiet time to practice. I arranged a room with space and growing plants and a sense of separateness; there I went on every morning. I read books on meditation, and from what I read I evolved my own practice. I also attended a Zen Center, spent some time in a Tibetan Buddhist retreat, and read deeply in the literature of Buddhism. In the end what evolved was my own way of being quiet. As I practiced, it became easier to quiet my mind, and I experienced a growing sense of calm and relaxation which I was often able to carry with me as I went about my daily life. The practice also increased my realization of what the inner world indeed was and I found that going there was a source of comfort and strength.

As I write this in 1977, I am aware that in spite of periods of discouragement and sadness, my sense of purpose and joyousness has grown. I am actively engaged in training for another career, and I have found many new friends. I am also aware that people around me want to know how it is with me. They ask "How are you?" and I realize that they want to be reassured that I am indeed well. But also I think, if the outcome had been different, I would still have something to bear witness to, that the choice of alternatives has a clarifying effect on one's attitude to life, and that whatever the result, it is possible to deepen one's inner life through meditation and to grow in the ability to meet whatever may eventuate . . . life or death.[35]

There are thus many reasons for minimizing mutilation and dealing in open, honest fashion with the problems of the cancer. To feel whole, to feel oneself as a woman, brings comfort not anguish, breeds peace not torment. One's whole life is beset with a succession of anxieties. Identifying each, not hiding them, enables a woman to master fears that are otherwise without limit. This applies to every phase of a long fight, but particularly at the end, when denial may cut a woman off from the warm human support that she most needs. So will she have peace of mind.

Though peace of mind in itself could be considered enough, there is something more: the influence of peace on immunity.[36] We have reason to believe that for many women, peace extends to the functions of the body, helping the struggles against invasion of the cancer — not a childish notion but a true force for good — peace, comfort, and well-being.

Chapter 12

The Shifting Emphasis in Diagnosis and Treatment

THIS CHAPTER is addressed to those of you who either are having some trouble with one of your breasts or who are concerned that trouble may occur. I shall discuss step by step the processes of making a diagnosis, what you should expect of your physician, and the treatment if treatment indeed is needed. First, a few reminders.

An age-old aphorism used by physicians in teaching medical students is that treatment of disease depends on three things: the first is the diagnosis; the second, the diagnosis; and the third, the diagnosis. It is a terse way of saying that once the diagnosis is established the treatment is clear, or if the diagnosis is fuzzy so too the treatment.

Among troubles of the breast, cancers are clearly the central problem. Numerically, however, they are a small problem. Cancers afflict at most 7 percent of women in the United States; at least 93 percent of you will never develop breast cancer.[1,2,3]

In contrast to cancers, other troubles of the breast are much more frequent. At least 50 percent of you, at one or another time during the active phase of your ovarian life, will have some lumpiness, that of the fibrocystic changes.[4] These changes would pass unnoticed were it not that the lumps of gland and fibrous tissue and cysts may mimic cancer. A major problem for you and your physicians, then, is to differentiate between these common changes and a rare cancer.

The benign neoplasms of the breast, the solid fibromas and fibroadenomas, are even less common than cancers, but because they may also resemble a malignant lesion they, too, must be identified and dealt with. In other words, even though cancers are uncommon, all lumps must be viewed with suspicion.

Cancer starts in one spot and grows out from that spot in all directions within the breast. It is therefore felt in its early phases as a localized lesion or lump and in one breast only.

If the cancer occurs in a breast that has no other identifiable lumps, the discovery and identification of the tumor are relatively easy. This is the condition of most women's breasts after the menopause, when glandular tissue of the breasts has atrophied and been replaced by fat.

If the cancer grows in a breast that is lumpy from fibrocystic changes — and we know the fibrocystic disorder is a condition many women have — then the determination of the type of the lump is immediately more difficult.

Lumps may be found by the woman herself, by a physician at a time of general examination, or by the routine application of tests, such as thermography and mammography.[5,6] As conditions are today, the majority of lumps, at least 80 percent, are picked up by the woman herself. This proportion may be expected to increase in the near future, as self-examination is practiced by more women. Even in the absence of a lump, there are other signals from the breast that should send a woman to her doctor.

Unusual pain or an area of unusual tenderness, a change in the pattern of discomfort associated with the menstrual cycle, should be checked if it persists after the period — even if you cannot find a lump. Persistence of pain in one area rarely points to a cancer, but is common in a developing cyst.

A change in size or shape of one breast, or a change in an area of one breast, either larger or smaller, should also be checked. This again is most likely the result of fibrocystic changes, but is not to be dismissed as being nothing. This is why you are supposed to watch your breasts in a mirror as you raise your arms: to notice if any area reacts differently from the comparable area in the opposite breast.

A retraction of a hitherto normal nipple or flaking of the nipple skin may indicate the development of a sluggish cancer of the ducts beneath the nipple or of the nipple itself.

Nipple discharge is also to be reported to your doctor. Unimportant is the small amount of clear fluid that many women have. The thing to take action on is a greater amount of discharge, particularly if it is bloody, which indicates some trouble in a duct.

When your doctor examines you he will repeat many of the steps of your own examination. Not only does he note what you have found, but he looks throughout both breasts for other lumpy areas. His examination may give him sufficient information to stop here. If he has any doubts, he may advise further studies. These may include thermography, mammography, aspiration of a lump with needle and syringe to see if it is a cyst, a needle biopsy, and, finally, excision of the lump to be sure of its nature (the excisional biopsy).[5,6,7,8]

All of these tests are used to make sure that a malignant condition is not present, or is promptly treated if it is present. Never forget that the big statistical likelihood is that any lump found is not malignant.

On the rare occasion that a malignancy seems to be present, the doctor will promptly order a bone scan, x-ray of the chest, blood studies, and other tests. These tests are made to determine if the cancer has already spread to distant organs of the body, principally bones, lungs, and liver.

At this point your physician will also want to know more about what is happening in the breast. He may advise studies by thermography and mammography.[5,6] Thermography registers changes in blood flow within the breast by measuring heat, and although it picks up those cancers with an increased blood flow, it also gives a positive shadow in many benign conditions, including the lumps of the fibrocystic disorder. Fibrocystic lumps are not all equally active metabolically, and therefore have differing blood flows. Some will show up, others not; and false positives are likely. Only if a single hot area shows up will thermography be helpful. Even so, this single area will need further identification. Because of false positives many doctors do not consider thermography worthwhile. On the other hand, the procedure does not harm the breast.

X-ray mammography, particularly Xeromammography, is the next step. It is the most reliable nonsurgical diagnostic test available. Now widely used as a screening procedure, it is unquestionably useful. It is so sharp that it may pick up a small malignant lesion that cannot be felt by the woman or the physician.

Unfortunately, mammography exposes the breasts to x-ray, and x-ray, even the small amount needed for the Xerogram, if repeated too often may theoretically harm the breasts. For a woman under 25, the chance of carcinoma is so unlikely, Xeromammography should be avoided as a routine. Only if a single lump persists is the x-ray exposure to be accepted at this age. If the woman is between 25 and 35, an occasional Xeromammogram is reasonable when a lump has been felt and its character has not been identified by needle aspiration. From the time the woman is 40, when cancer appears with increasing frequency, the Xeromammogram is indicated whenever the nature of a lump is in doubt. It should preferably not be used as a routine screening device, like the vaginal smear, until women are past 50 — and then only annually.

If the character of the lump and the mammogram suggest that the lump is a cyst, simple aspiration of the fluid by a needle and syringe is the most direct and helpful diagnostic test. Any fluid aspirated is, of course, examined by the pathologist for possible cells.[8]

If the lump proves to be solid — that is, if it has no fluid in it — the physician may then advise a needle biopsy.[7] A needle larger than the aspirating needle, with a sharp cutting point, cuts a core as it passes through the tumor. It is a test recommended by some physicians, but its use depends upon the availability of an especially versed pathologist, and only a few physicians have such experts to call on. The absence of cancer cells does not conclusively mean that the tumor is benign.

If these needle maneuvers do not give a definite answer, or if the necessary pathological work is not available, the physician will want to take out the whole lump, just to be sure of what is going on. This is called a "surgical biopsy." Unfortunately, this procedure leaves a scar, but it can be done in a manner to disturb the contour of the breast as little as possible.

Now back to your lump.

The most common condition giving rise to lumps, as we already know, is the fibrocystic disorder. We presume that this is the condition you have. You are therefore in the premenopausal years. (We shall deal later with the troubles of the postmenopausal woman.) With this disorder we also know the following: that the lumps are multiple, of the same general character, and evenly distributed throughout both breasts.

Because you have so many, you and your doctor will discuss the lessened likelihood of any one of the lumps' being malignant.

Because the lumps in all probability are not malignant, your doctor may well advise you to watch them through at least one, perhaps two, menstrual cycles, to see if they all wax and wane in characteristic fashion. If most do but one does not, then that one is something different, out of line, and calls for further study.

The Xeromammogram the physician orders may be expected to reveal not only fibrous tissue exaggeration, but also overgrowths of the gland and ductal cells. The radiologist terms these "sclerosing adenosis" and "ductal dysplasia." These cell exaggerations are no more threatening than that of the fibrous tissue, but knowing of their presence is helpful to both surgeon and pathologist should a biopsy be needed later on. Cysts and unexpected small neoplasms, benign and malignant, may of course be revealed. If all lumpy areas cast equal shadows, and nothing suggesting a neoplasm is seen to confirm the physical examination, the doctor will understandably advise watchful waiting — re-examination after two cycles and periodic checks every three to six months, according to your age and the degree of the physician's suspicion.

The function of the ovaries and the condition of the uterus are to be considered. The same ovarian hormones stimulate both the uterus and breasts. If there has been a change — even a slight change — in the monthly cycles, and if the uterus is larger than anticipated for a woman of your age and the lining of the uterus (the endometrium) is hyperplastic, these signs offer helpful confirmation that the changes in the breasts are caused by the fibrocystic disorder.

If this lump you have found differs from the other lumps, it's a different ball game; something else is happening. The most likely diagnosis is a cyst. If it has a smooth capsule and, particularly, if it waxes and wanes or has appeared in a woman in her 40s during a month or two without a period, the doctor may proceed immediately, without a mammogram, to tap it with a needle and syringe.

If it has a thick fibrous capsule, a cyst may feel irregular, more like a cancerous growth. The mammogram may show it as a rounded, smooth, encapsulated mass. In this case also, the physician may try to aspirate the mass with needle and syringe.

If he encounters fluid and empties the cyst, the mass usually disappears. The physician then sends the aspirated fluid to the pathologist to look for cells that may be floating in it. An occasional cyst has a malignant lining, the fluid being a secretion of a special cancer, sometimes a papillary malignancy of low invasive character. If cells in the fluid are of such a nature, subsequent excision of the lump with a generous margin of the surrounding uninvolved normal breast is all the treatment that tumor needs.

If the aspirated fluid contains no cells or only benign cells, well and good.

If the needle tap obtained no fluid, the tumor presumably is solid.

The doctor can tell a lot as he passes the needle into one side, through the tumor, and out the far side. If the tumor is solid, it is presumably a neoplasm. If you are a younger woman, 18 to 25, it may well be a benign fibroma or adenofibroma. If so, there is no hurry. But the neoplasm will grow and have to be removed eventually; it may be removed soon, at a convenient time. Then the correct diagnosis will be assured and anxiety reduced. The removal will, however, leave a scar.

If you are a woman in your 40s when fibromas are rare, some doctors will advocate needle biopsy for a definitive diagnosis. As in a younger woman, the more certain step, and probably the wiser policy, is to have the entire tumor excised. In this way, again, the possibility of a cancer is excluded and calm has a chance to return.

If the evidence regarding the isolated lump suggests that it may be malignant — that is, if needle aspiration proves it to be solid (particularly if the needle grated as it was passed through the tumor), if a needle biopsy was done and is suggestive of cancer, if the Xeromammogram shows a cluster of minute calcifications or a spreading shadow where the tumor is felt — then an excisional biopsy is prudent, on the assumption that it is cancer. If your lump proves to be cancer, treatment must follow, as indicated below under Care of Cancer.

Do not be alarmed by needle aspirations, needle biopsies, or even excisional biopsies; all can be done under so-called local anesthesia. The only pain you will notice is that of the fine needle used to inject the anesthetic. If you understand what is contemplated, the little pain of the injection is tolerable. The use of the local anesthesia, with you awake, is far preferable to having you put to sleep for such short procedures, but you can plan this with your physician beforehand.

Care of Recurrent Cysts. If the studies have excluded a fibroma or a carcinoma, you, the patient, are still left with the fibrocystic disorder, the nature of which you should understand fully.

Recurrent cysts may continue to be a problem right up to, and into the time of, your menopause. The fluid in the majority of cysts goes away by itself, but sometimes the fluid continues to collect and the cyst remains tender, a source of annoyance and worry. Aspiration usually ends the story, but occasionally the cyst may refill. If it refills repeatedly, then it may be helpful to have it taken out. This is rarely necessary.

Too often cysts are removed because the doctor is worried about the diagnosis, and, as we have seen, the diagnosis can usually be arrived at by simpler measures. Cysts just have to be kept after, and care has to be taken by the physician that a malignant type of tumor does not develop nearby and be mistaken for the cyst.

Other than the above reason, the fibrocystic disorder is not basically a worrisome condition, uncomfortable though it may be at times. It is not a contraindication to the Pill or to a pregnancy — indeed, pregnancy will relieve the condition — and it is not a significant precursor of cancer. Its continued presence, however, may be a source of worry, and it is also a matter of concern in the use of female hormones as a pre- and post-menopausal therapy. We will deal more with these aspects in Chapter 13.

Care of Cancer. In the care of the malignant neoplasms, there are several principles to be kept in mind. First, there are at least fifteen different types of breast cancer, from sluggish, barely invasive tumors to highly malignant, widely spreading cancers.[9,10,11] For the sluggish growth, simple excision, which distorts the breast as little as possible, is adequate therapy. For the highly malignant ones, all available therapies are needed: surgery, radiation, and drugs. Second, it is to be emphasized that there are new outlooks, new hopes; not just better radiation and more powerful drugs, but immunotherapy is on the horizon. The progress in cancer research is rapid, and with each new piece of knowledge, there is a new chance for effective therapy. Care has improved enormously in the last five years, and hope is increasing even more for the next few years. It is a time of excitement and achievement. Our recommendations must take this progress into account.

Foremost among the new knowledge that is changing our emphasis is the realization of the early widespread dissemination of cancer cells in the majority of patients currently being encountered in the United States. This dissemination must have occurred before the patient first found her lump and before any therapy had been carried out. No matter how good any operation, or combination of limited operation and primary irradiation, is in eliminating the cancer from the breast and breast region, this regional treatment fails to cure the disease. It is essential to point out that the majority of patients must receive additional therapy for the widespread disease. Although no better at saving life than the older mastectomies, limited excision and primary radiation do spare a woman unnecessary mutilation and crippling of arm and shoulder.

I have inveighed against radical mastectomy; indeed, against any operation that removes the entire breast. The radical operation fails to cure the majority of patients because it does not reach the cancer cells that have passed elsewhere in the body. The minority of patients whom the operation does cure have a sluggish, confined cancer, and a simpler, less mutilating operation would be sufficient. Since the alternative treatment of a limited excision, with minimal distortion of the breast plus primary radiation to the residual breast, is equally effective in eradicating cancer cells from the breast and breast region — and since this alternative treatment is far less mutilating and easier for a woman to bear — radical surgical operations should be a thing of the past.

I have also been emphasizing the use of antitumor drugs. These are effective against many, even if not all, breast cancers. They offer much beyond the palliative endocrine maneuvers that have been emphasized over so many years. These drugs provide the first hope of cure rather than of mere delay.

The pathologist's growing appreciation of the biologic nature of the several breast cancers is of increasing importance. The arrival of the antitumor drugs has forced this more detailed study upon us. The medical profession has been slow to appreciate that the clinical state or stage of the disease at the time the woman is first seen is not nearly so important as knowing the true biologic nature of the tumor. Drugs are toxic and should not be given heedlessly to all patients. Those whose cancers are localized within the breast and have been eradicated by surgery, irradiation, or a combination of both will not need the drugs. We must emphasize that the time has arrived when we *can* differentiate between those who need all therapies and those who can be adequately cared for with a simpler treatment.

A comprehensive program of therapy has therefore evolved out of our experience of the past five years.[11] There are four steps to this program: surgery, pathology, radiotherapy, and chemotherapy.

The first step is surgical and has the following six elements:

1. The diagnosis is established by means of the surgical biopsy described above.

2. The entire gross tumor is removed in order to eliminate the bulk of the tumor cells, thus reducing the dose of radiation should subsequent irradiation be needed.

3. The tumor is removed with its capsule so that, if it proves to be noninvasive or only sluggishly invasive, a second, more extended operation will not be needed.

4. Your surgeon should remove enough of the surrounding apparently uninvolved breast in order to give the pathologist a sufficiently clear picture of how the tumor is spreading. But if the tumor is invasive, irradiation of the entire residual breast will be needed, and nothing will have been gained by a halfway measure. (The tumor removal is not intended to take care of the dissemination into other parts of your breast; radiation will take care of this.)

5. A biopsy of the lower axillary lymph nodes is indicated through either the incision already made or a small, second direct one.

6. Your breast should be distorted as little as possible, if the surgeon excises only that amount of breast consistent with the above surgical objectives.

Finally, after operation, your breast is snugly bound in an elastic adhesive brassiere with a bountiful gauze dressing. Your surgeon will have been careful to tie all the little blood vessels, so drainage of the wound will not be necessary.

The Pathologist's Inning. At the close of the operation, the pathologist has the entire gross tumor, some surrounding breast tissue, and the lower axillary lymph nodes. He now needs time for a detailed study of the tumor to determine the character of the cells and the nature of their spread. We have to have this information to know how to treat you, the patient. If the tumor proves to be noninvasive, the limited excision already done will suffice. If it is invasive, and 90 percent are, the breast will need to be irradiated. Depending on the character of the invasion, the regional lymph nodes may also need irradiation, and if the invasion indicates widespread dissemination, chemotherapy should follow the irradiation.

The pathologist grades the cells as to their invasive potential, the rate of growth as shown by the number of mitotic figures, and the manner in which the cells invade other tissues, including the blood and lymphatic vessels and nerve sheaths. For the delineation of blood vessel invasion alone, elastic tissue stains are required, and these take two days. Invasions of the lymphatic vessels and nerve sheaths are important; they point to a tumor of more than average virulence. The margin of the tumor is inspected for the fibrous pushing margin and/or lymphocytic infiltrate. These two signs of host resistance are important in the decision regarding chemotherapy and the choice of the drugs.

Little of this information essential to your care as a patient can be seen by the pathologist on the frozen section preparation. All the information that the frozen section can yield is whether cancer is present or not. The frozen section interpretation, as we learned earlier, is sometimes subject to misdiagnosis, particularly in regard to the cellular sclerosing adenosis of the fibrocystic disorder. The traditional surgical custom of requesting the pathologist to give a frozen section diagnosis while the patient is still on the operating table, still under anesthesia, and then proceeding immediately to radical mastectomy if the pathologist reports cancer is no longer acceptable; it can lead to inadequate information and the occasional error of a diagnosis of cancer when, in fact, no cancer exists.

A designation as to the type of breast cancer present is essential to your continual care. Older classification systems no longer suffice. We now find that of Ackerman to be the most useful.[9,10] His Types indicate the appropriate sequence of treatments.

Ackerman's Type I cancers are localized *in situ* cancers (5 to 10 percent of breast cancers). They are noninvasive, and the excision of the tumor with an adequate margin is all the treatment needed. No radiation; no drugs.

Type II cancers are somewhat more malignant; the cells have managed to penetrate the surrounding membrane and are invading slowly out into the rest of the breast (10 to 15 percent of breast cancers). These tumors are adequately treated by removal of the lump followed by irradiation of the remaining breast. The lymph nodes are not involved and nothing is gained by irradiating them. Chemotherapy is not needed since there are no cells widespread through the body.

Type III cancers are move invasive (35 to 45 percent of breast cancers). In general, the cells have spread into the lymph nodes as well as throughout the breast. For both breast and nodes, irradiation will be needed. It can also safely be assumed, in this type, that cells have become widely dispersed throughout the body and chemotherapy will be needed promptly and for long periods. The chemotherapy is advised even though no cancer cells can be demonstrated in bones by bone scan, lungs by x-rays, or liver by chemical tests or scan.

The Type IV cancers are the most virulent (35 to 45 percent of breast cancers). All of those that invade blood vessels are included in this group. So are those in which the cells are rapidly dividing and are distributed through the breast and beyond, into the chest wall and the skin. As with patients who have Type III cancers, irradiation is given to the breast and breast region, followed by chemotherapy. Of all the cancers, these need the most prompt and prolonged drug therapy.

Without the pathologist's detailed information about type, treatment at best is fuzzy and frequently illogical. There is no sense, to take the extreme example, in treating a patient with a Type I cancer as if she had Type IV disease, irradiating her breast and giving her drugs that she does not need. Or the reverse, treating a patient with a Type IV cancer as if she had a Type I tumor, failing to give her the radiation and drugs so necessary for her future well-being. No longer can we be satisfied with one treatment for all; radical mastectomy for everybody. Full information is essential to modern progressive care.

With the pathologist's designation of type of cancer, your diagnosis is established and treatment begins. As treatment starts, you have the right to choose between radical surgery and primary irradiation. Many doctors will continue to advise radical mastectomy or one of its modifications. And those of you who have confidence in your physician should feel free to accept the operative treatment — provided you understand and are ready for the possible shock from the loss of the breast, and for possible hindrance to the motion of shoulder and arm. As far as getting rid of the cancer cells in the breast itself, the operation is as good as the radiation. You should remember also that if lymph nodes are involved, the radical operation removes only those nodes in the axilla, and leaves the treatment of those in front and back of the chest to radiation.

On the other hand, those patients among you who choose the primary radiation should recall that this must be a full tumor dose, not a lesser adjuvant dose. Radiotherapists will have different views as to just how the several breast areas should be treated and by what instruments. They will want to tie together their treatment with what was seen by the pathologist. You will be unwise to ask for a shorter treatment period, since this might well mean a lesser total dose. You should remember that there are reasons for dividing the treatment into several small doses, covering at least five, perhaps, better, six or seven, weeks.

There are also decisions to be made by the radiotherapist regarding the lymph nodes involved. The nodes should be watched carefully in case the nature of the dissemination was not apparent in the microscopic sections. If enlarged lymph nodes should eventually appear, they can be irradiated at that later time. Present evidence indicates that little will have been lost by the waiting.

In patients with Type II, III, or IV cancers there is no question that the nodes should be treated, and presumably those in all four areas. Some radiotherapists may feel that if the cancer was in that portion of the breast tucked right up underneath the arm, then the axillary are the only nodes needing treatment. And, conversely, if the cancer lay toward the middle of the chest, then only the nodes under the sternum should be treated. It would be helpful for you to know that the radiotherapist had consulted with the pathologist about the probable distribution of the cancer cells in the nodes.

The full tumor dose of radiation will inevitably result in some temporary reddening of the skin, resembling sunburn. Occasionally, blisters will form, as they do following a severe sunburn; but they will dry up spontaneously and the reddening will disappear, a little more slowly than a sunburn, but disappear it will. As it disappears there may well be slight pigmentation; this, too, will fade, as a summer tan fades.

Once the radiation has been finished and the scarlet reaction has subsided, the chemotherapy should be started for patients with Type III or IV cancer. Differences of opinion regarding the drugs to be used and the duration of treatment are to be expected. In the next few years, evidence will be forthcoming regarding specificity of certain drugs for certain cancers. We know now that some cancers are sensitive to hormones and others are not, and it is only reasonable to anticipate comparable differences in sensitivity to drugs.

We don't know this, but it is also reasonable to suppose that cancer cells at first sensitive to a drug will become resistant to it. Therefore, drugs should be changed from time to time and alternated. In any event, at the present time we consider multiple drugs advisable, and two years a minimum for the drug program.

Obviously, as the patient, you should be fully informed regarding such possible sensitivity reactions to drugs as nausea, loss of hair, or the cessation of menstrual periods. You should notify your physician at the earliest appearance of such signs so that the drugs can be promptly changed.

The comprehensive program (limited surgery, irradiation, and chemotherapy) also cares for the special situations of multicentric foci and bilateral cancers. The multicentric foci in the breast harboring the major cancer will have been destroyed by the irradiation, and any such foci in the opposite breast will undoubtedly be attacked by the chemotherapy and presumably handled in this manner. The initial physical examination and mammographic studies will have excluded the presence of a second cancer in the opposite breast, but it is, of course, possible that a minute second cancer, too small to be recognized, has already started. Here again, the prompt drug therapy will attack this second cancer as well as distant foci, and theoretically will be as effective as the drugs are against any other cancer focus.

You and your physician should set up periodic follow-up examinations. These will call for the physician to observe the disappearance of the original cancer or its possible resurgence. Also, a second cancer may appear in the later years. (This happens in approximately 7 percent of patients who have had one breast cancer.) Follow-up, therefore, keeps on indefinitely. As you yourself learn the several problems you face, you will take on an increasing part of the follow-up, with fewer mandatory visits to your physician. (The follow-up visits should be a part of the periodic general examinations that include Pap smear, blood pressure measurement, tests for anemia, diabetes, and like diseases).

From time to time, despite all efforts, there will be patients with progressive, demonstrable disease in bones, lungs, and liver. In some of you, this may be apparent when you are first seen; in others, this may appear later despite the treatment to breast and lymph nodes. Those among you who have not had any treatment to your breast should at least have the tumor removed so that the dissemination of cells is cut down. All should be treated for the far-flung disease. As we know, much can be done, both by drugs and endocrine maneuvers, to establish a holding pattern.

There may well be differences of opinion among physicians as to which attack to launch first. Some will favor immediate endocrine change, either by removing the ovaries or by giving estrogens. If you are one of the 30 to 40 percent who benefit, the endocrine maneuvers should be pursued one after another, the ultimate being the irradiation of the pituitary gland. Much comfort can be obtained by these endocrine changes, and they are not to be lightly dismissed.

Other physicians will prefer immediate drug treatment, leaving the endocrine maneuvers in reserve. Here again, if there is pain, comfort is restored and much can be achieved over a period of years. With both endocrine and drug treatment available, you and your family should not despair.

Even as you read this, new knowledge will have come, bringing advances in treatment. Fewer cancers will persist; more will have been eradicated; and newer methods of treating the widespread lesions (in the form of more effective drugs) will have arrived upon the scene.

I have not dealt here with sarcomas and other rare tumors, and I have not discussed the differential diagnosis of infections. Infections in the lactation period or later, at the time of the menopause, often cause local inflammation or small abscesses resembling malignant tumors. There is also a poorly understood condition called "fat necrosis," in which a fatty area in the breast develops a noninfectious inflammation simulating a malignant tumor on physical examination. These are now more easily differentiated from cancer by the mammographic techniques, but still they give trouble and have to be thought of constantly. Areas of fat necrosis are also difficult to distinguish from the cancer on frozen section, which is another reason why the pathologist must be given sufficient time to establish the diagnosis with certainty.*

This is not all. There are the long stretches after treatment, and the need for you and your doctor to keep in touch. No matter how well things are going, there are, inevitably, abrupt emotional crises — a friend whose cancer has returned, a shadow in

*In this account thus far, the descriptions of diagnosis and treatment have been cut to the bone, giving only that information needed for the immediate care of the woman with a lumpy breast. The specific references for the diagnostic measures and several treatments are, for the most part, given in the individual chapters describing the biology of the breast, tumors, surgery, radiation, hormones, chemotherapy, and immunotherapy. These will be considered further in the final chapter.

the lung due perhaps to viral pneumonia, not to a return of the cancer. Your doctor and you each need a sense of balance and perspective to live through such interruptions.

If the disease comes back and grows beyond control, while there are yet enormous opportunities for help, the time comes when medical measures are no longer useful and extreme treatments can be harmful, disturbing to everybody. The Reach to Recovery program is not appropriate to this phase of life. Still, much can be done. The Make Today Count organization has proven a boon to many. Dr. Elisabeth Kübler-Ross gives extraordinarily good advice in her book *On Death and Dying*. Both of these sources of help are cited in the Appendix.

Chapter 13

Good Care, Now and in the Future

THROUGHOUT THIS BOOK I have spoken out against surgical removal of the breast, against radical mastectomy, modified radical, or mastectomy in any form. I have spoken not because removal is harmful in the treatment of the cancer, but because such operations are disfiguring, thoughtless of woman's feelings about herself, and damaging to her emotional well-being. Seventy-five and fifty years ago, when there was no alternative to surgical treatment, doctors and women had to turn their backs to the harm that was being inflicted. But now, with our understanding of the complexity of the disease, of how it spreads, and with the development of radiation techniques and successful drug therapy, there are alternatives.

For many years a few physicians in the United States and Canada have agreed that, as far as the care of the cancer is concerned, limited excision of the tumor followed by irradiation to the remaining breast offers as good care as any of the operations removing the breast.[1-4]

In recent years several more physicians, particularly radiotherapists, have supported the less mutilating program.[5-8] But it must be stressed that, at the present writing, the vast majority of physicians, particularly surgeons, adhere to the traditional surgical program of mastectomy in one form or another.[9] Many of these same physicians are concerned about the dangers of radiotherapy and of the possible consequences of drug therapy.[10]

Because of this continued adherence to the traditional treatment, the woman who wishes to consider the new approach is almost certain to find opposition among the doctors she consults. Her physicians may conscientiously consider it far from wise to bank on the new and untried, to neglect the tried and proven. Many doctors have a way of putting aside questions that imply criticism of their traditional point of view. After all, traditional treatment in a sense protects the physician. It keeps him from making an error in the care of his patients. As long as he follows traditional practice, he knows he has done the right thing and is safe from criticism or suit.

There will also be practical problems. Even if her family physician is sympathetic, a woman may encounter difficulty in finding a surgeon who will agree that a limited excision of a tumor is reasonable. He may feel he would be doing her harm by such an operation. In this case, what does she do? Where does she go?

Too, there may not be a radiotherapist experienced in primary irradiation of the breast. How large a dose is needed to cure? Will such a dose lead to disfigurement? The United States is huge. Although in 1974 there were 1500 cobalt machines, and more have been added since that time, still the presence of the machine is not in itself sufficient.[11] A woman needs a radiologist specially trained in therapy, and these are still in short supply.

She may find it difficult to get the needed advice about other of the special problems. Not all physicians are prepared to examine her breasts or even to make a pelvic examination. These other areas relate not only to her general health, but also quite specifically to the care of her breasts.

Cancer is but one aspect. The benign breast lumps, the problems of the female hormone in the Pill and at the menopause, mammograms, and many other things recur throughout a woman's life.

Life is complicated; so is medicine. Medicine has met its complexity by specializations; its vast knowledge is divided into many areas. In present-day medicine, the breast is cared for by the general surgeon, the ovaries by the gynecologist, the thyroid by the thyroidologist, and the function of the brain by the psychiatrist and neurologist. Other specialists are called upon to care for an upset stomach, pneumonia, or kidney trouble. No matter how kindly and considerate the family doctor is, he is put to it to cover all these fields of expertise. If the specialists are available, a woman is all too soon divided up into special compartments of care. Not infrequently, she may receive conflicting advice from these several specialists. How is she to find her way through this maze of special knowledge?

What does a woman need a doctor for? First, he may be consulted about the development of her breasts — are they too small or too large — matters of enormous psychological import. Then, there are the diffuse lumps of the cyclic changes and the localized lumps, both benign and malignant. These lumps cover woman's life span from puberty through old age. If we are not careful in our planning, the examination of the breasts becomes an enormous burden.

Self-examination. Since the majority of cancers are picked up by the women themselves, the American Cancer Society, the American College of Obstetricians and Gynecologists, and many physicians recommend that women examine their breasts themselves as a routine. By this recommendation, it is hoped, more cancers will be picked up early, when treatment is more secure and successful. The recommendation is, of course, a wise one but it is not just off-hand easy. The woman must learn how and when to make the examination. Some doctors emphasize that breast self-examination should start in adolescence and continue every month throughout life. Others suggest that women start at age 30 and make the examination only twice a year. What is best?

A sense of proportion is essential, and each woman should aim at developing a program on her own. I shall begin with an absurd statistic. If breast self-examination is recommended for every young woman, starting at age 18 or 20, her younger sister, aged 14, whose breasts are developing, will want to start breast self-examination also. It is the thing to do! Suppose the 14-

year-old sister examines her breasts every month until she is 74, the present average survival age of women. For such a woman it would mean 12 examinations for each of fifty years, a total of 720 examinations. Supposing that 100 young women entered such a program; that would mean 72,000 examinations. Since only 7 of these 100 women may be expected to develop cancer, it would mean that 10,286 self-examinations would be performed to pick up one cancer. Inherent in such a number of examinations lies the danger that the examinations would become perfunctory. An examination repeated over and over again with negative results may become less thorough. The examination is better not made if not painstakingly done.

I use these absurd figures to illustrate the problem. In order to get any one of us to do something like breast self-examination, we have to be reminded about what may happen if we don't. Such a reminder may be frightening and could interfere with a woman's whole life and her attitude toward health. The thought about possible cancer has to be tempered with reason. It is part of the perspective. In terms of what we know today, this is what I advise.

It is helpful to all women to know that, as they go through life, it is normal for changes to occur in their breasts. In Chapter 5 we saw that of young women aged 20 to 30, only 2 per 100,000 develop cancer in any one year. That is the age group in which there is a peak of fibrocystic changes. Lots and lots of lumps will be felt and will need to be identified. Since the incidence of cancer is so low, self-examination need not be carried out any more often than every six months; for example, January and July. It should be carried out at the same phase in the ovarian cycle, preferably one week after the onset of menstruation, when the breasts should be the most quiescent. (See the Appendix, pages 199–206, including the diagrams of the American College of Obstetricians and Gynecologists. They are good.) At one or two visits to her doctor, she should check to be sure her skill in self-examination is perfected.

X-ray mammograms are most useful and helpful in the diagnosis of a lump.[12] They are probably less useful in screening out dangerous lumps in women in whom no lump can be felt by herself or by her doctor. Since there is no doubt that exposure to x-rays can be injurious to tissues, and particularly to the tissues of the young, mammograms in women under 50 should be taken only after due thought. This means that they should not be taken as a routine annual test by women below the age of 50. But if a lump has been identified, no matter what the woman's age — 18, 20, 30, or 40 — then a mammogram may be a reasonable step.[13]

Annual Health Examination. Beginning at age 16, each woman will do wisely to seek an annual health examination. The examination will include, besides a general physical, a check of the breasts, uterus, and ovaries. The Pap smear can also give important information regarding ovarian function. It is not limited to testing for cancer of the uterus or cervix, and should therefore be included in a general examination. The taking of a Pap smear should certainly start after the woman has begun bearing children, or when she is in her 30s in any case. (The routine mammogram comes later, in the 50s.) The function of the thyroid, too, must be considered because of the relation of low thyroid function to continued secretion of milk and, occasionally, to cancer.[14]

There are many more things important to a woman's breasts and to health than just the annual examination: avoidance of polluted environments, particularly if she plans to have a child; her diet, rest, and sleep; a sense of being in charge of her life. For most of this she must take the responsibility. For much of this she does not need a doctor.

I have referred throughout to the Pill and other uses of estrogen hormone in treatment, and its relation to fibrocystic changes. A few reminders are pertinent.

There is no question about the Pill. It's a boon to society and can sometimes be effective therapy for women with excessive fibrocystic changes.

Use of estrogen for eternal youth requires large doses and carries some risk, maybe not great. The woman herself has to decide. I cannot in all conscience recommend such use.

The use of small doses of estrogen for hot flashes and other symptoms of the menopause is a godsend to some women, but such use is not needed forever, and many women never need it at all. It should not, therefore, be routine following a hysterectomy or the natural menopause. A vaginal cream containing a small dose of estrogens is often useful to maintain the moisture and elasticity of the vagina.

There is one use of the estrogen hormone mandatory for some women. It has long been known that the bones of women past the menopause are more easily broken than those of men of the same age. In childhood there is no difference in the incidence of broken bones between girls and boys. From childhood on, there is a very slow increase in the number of fractures in both men and women. After the age of 50 this slow rise continues for men; but women, in contrast, have an abrupt increase, particularly fractures of the hip and arm. The bones of some women begin to thin out and lose strength after the change of life, and if they fall, their bones are more likely to break.

This thinning of women's bones has been extensively investigated.[15-18] The strength of the bones of women and the maintenance of that strength after the menopause follow an ethnic pattern. Black-skinned women lose the least amount of bone strength. Brown- and yellow-skinned women are only mildly affected. It is white women with unpigmented skin who suffer the most. One third of white women are not noticeably affected. One-third suffer a moderate loss of bone strength but are little troubled by the loss. The final third undergo material loss of bone mass and strength. The majority of these last, or one fourth of the total of white women, suffer bone fractures or significant bone pain.

It has been found that a small dose of estrogen hormone given daily, starting at the menopause, prevents this deterioration of bone strength. In Caucasian women in whom use of the estrogen is delayed for five to ten years after the menopause, the

hormone stops the progress of the thinning but it does not always restore the original strength. It is therefore of importance
to women with unpigmented skin that the group into which
they fall be established early after the change of life. At approximately 50, or at the menopause if that comes earlier, they
should have the strength of their bones standardized by an x-ray
and the course of their bone strength carefully followed for the
next few years. At the earliest sign of loss of strength, estrogen
hormones should be instituted. Obviously, it is only for the one
woman in three who needs it. Fortunately, the dose of estrogen
required to maintain bone strength is a small one, not large
enough to interfere with the integrity of the lining of the uterus
or with the breast.[17]

No account of self-examination of the breasts and the fibrocystic lumps that are likely to be encountered is adequate without a
reminder of the role of the ovaries and how the ovaries are governed by the higher centers of the brain. Every woman learns at
some point that the cycle of her ovaries, normally regular at approximately twenty-eight days, may be disturbed one way or
another by some emotional trouble — a sick child, the death of a
parent, moving house and home, or an ecstatic event. Such
women will not be surprised to learn that at many colleges, as
many as 30 percent of freshmen women miss one or more of
their periods in the first months of the freshman year. These
missed periods are easy enough to understand. For many of
these young women, it is their first time away from home. They
come to a dormitory life with strange roommates, in strange surroundings, and all the time they are forced to meet new strin-
gent academic standards. A knowing health-service physician
does not think only of an unwanted pregnancy but can reassure
each young woman that her periods will no doubt return after
November examinations or at least when she comes back after
the Christmas vacation to surroundings that are by now familiar.

It is well understood how the emotional temper of the brain is
reflected in the action of the ovaries.[19] The immediate control of

the ovaries comes, as we have already learned, from the anterior pituitary gland lying at the base of the brain. The pituitary, in turn, is directed by the hypothalamus, the lowest part of the forebrain. The hypothalamus manages most of the automatic functions of the body, such as heartbeat, respiration, temperature control, and digestion. In addition to governing the ovaries, it controls most of the other endocrine glands. This area of the brain is of the lowest order common to all mammals. It is a part of the brain that does not think and has no discriminatory power.

Discrimination and change of function in response to unusual circumstances stem from the midbrain, above the hypothalamus, of which the limbic system is the most important part.[20] It sorts out the messages from our conscious gray matter and sends on what it judges appropriate to the automatic hypothalamus for action. It is where experience is stored, and has the capacity to make judgments even though we are not conscious of them. It is the part of the brain that tells the cat to get ready to jump into a tree if a dog appears. It recognizes the meaning of the dog when the eyes or nose or ears of the cat sense the approach of the dog. It digests the messages. If the senses observe a threatening situation, an alerting, alarming message is referred by the limbic system to the hypothalamus. In lower mammals, such as the cat or the dog, these messages are largely limited in variety to matters like hunger, sex, fear, anger, and joy at seeing its master. In the human being, the messages are of far greater variety and complexity, for they involve memory and the traditional ways of behavior. The need to make new friends in a strange, competitive environment may disturb the limbic system because it is unaccustomed to, and threatened by, such events. On the other hand, young women who have had successful earlier experiences may continue in the normal ovarian timetable undisturbed. So, too, in older women, the elation of the prospect of a new love relationship may reactivate earlier patterns of gland function. The following experiences of two women indicate how the limbic system may become involved!

A woman of 28 developed a lump in her breast that was needled without producing any fluid. It was therefore resected under local anesthesia. It proved to be an encapsulated benign fibroma. The lump had developed three years after the birth of her third and last child. It was a phase in her life when her breasts were regularly swollen and tender before her periods. In the succeeding years, the tenderness and swelling became less and less, the duration and flow of her periods increased. In her 42nd year she noticed that her periods had shortened and returned to the same character as when she was in her 20s. Concomitant with this change, she noticed the appearance of a lump in the opposite breast. She concluded that it was another fibroma. The doctor she contacted advised immediate excision, but she decided to wait over her next period before reporting to her surgeon. Immediately after the period, the lump disappeared. Two weeks later she came to see me, telling me of the change in her periods and the disappearance of the lump. She asked whether it could be that the reversal of her ovarian pattern had been initiated by the children's being grown and in college — flown the coop, so to speak. I suspected another reason for the changes. Obviously the lump must have been a cyst, for that is the only kind of a lump that could have vanished spontaneously. I knew that more than ten years ago she and her husband had separated. Surely now there was a reactivation of the ovarian cycle more like that of her fertile years. I told her, therefore, that more probably there had been a change in her sexual life. She said yes, my supposition was correct — a new suitor, a most attractive man, a new life ahead.

A woman of 46, healthy throughout her life, suddenly developed a nodule in one breast. Before its appearance, she had missed two periods. She was, of course, alarmed; perhaps it was a cancer. The first surgeon she consulted advised removal of the nodule to make sure. The second doctor aspirated the lump, removing clear fluid, thus answering the question of its nature. Her periods resumed, the cyst did not refill, and no new lumps have formed. The cyst had developed, no doubt, because of the sudden change in her periods. But why had she missed those two periods? At a number of times in her life, she had had ardent suitors. Suddenly a new suitor had appeared, an ideal person, and a new vision appeared on the horizon. That was why.

Fortunately these two women were able to tell me what was taking place in their lives and we, they and I, were not at a loss for explanation.

The central nervous system of the human being is enormously complex and I have been dealing only with one part, that part which integrates thought and the function of women's glands. This very complexity betokens the extraordinary capacity of the brain — the capacity for thought, reasoning, adjustment, adaptation, and survival, a capacity that distinguishes the human being from all other animals. There is no special strength in human bones compared with that in other animals, the dog or the cow. There is nothing special or unusual in human muscle or in the digestive tract or other organs. What men and women have accomplished, what they are able to do and withstand, is the result of the complexity and capacity of the brain.

It is also the complexity of the human brain that makes it so difficult for many of us to control our emotions and modify our patterns of thinking and living. Yet with determination we may be able to modify our outlook and our ways. If we can come to understand the anxieties and patterns of thought that limit our physical actions, we can lessen our worries, bring ourselves reassurance, calm, and new happiness.

Accomplishing change is often difficult to do alone. Many of us are helped by an advisor. In the past we have turned to older, wiser people. Now there are others — minister, priest, psychiatrist, nurse, and social worker.

The glandular system of women is far more complex than that of men. Women thus may confront greater difficulties; and yet, on the other hand, they have more to gain by restoring calm. But what must be understood at the beginning is that each woman, each individual, has the responsibility to maintain her health, to seek help wherever and whenever needed. Don't be afraid to ask; there is so much to be gained.

Urgency of Care. Doctors have long known that if they can identify and treat a disease early in its development, it is easier to eradicate. This applies to malignant tumors, pneumonia, typhoid fever, and many other diseases. For this reason, urgency has become part of the traditional care of cancer of the breast. The American Cancer Society is pleading for promptness, and it is unquestionably important. On the other hand, urgency may lead to false and unnecessary steps.

Prompt Reporting. The prompt reporting of a lump in the breast to the physician is sensible. Don't be railroaded, however, into immediate operation. If you find yourself under pressure, show your doctor this book and draw the notes and sources to his attention.

Most lumps are benign: 93 percent of women never develop cancer of the breast. And much the same is true of lumps of the uterus — uterine fibroids and cervical polyps. Any delay, however, must have a reason, something to gain and more than offset possible harm from waiting. If you wish to avoid unnecessary mutilation, refuse to sign the hospital form that gives blanket permission for a radical mastectomy while you are asleep. The delay will give you time to hear the results of the biopsy and enter into the decision regarding further treatment. And it won't hurt. It is your right.

For Those Who Have Had a Radical Mastectomy. To those of you who may already have had a radical mastectomy, or those who have a relative or friend who has had one, I can say that I am sure your doctor did the best that he knew how. I am not saying that your operation was wrong at the time it was carried out. In terms of cancer care, the operation was a good one. But you should now find out whether you need chemotherapy. If there was any chance that cells might have spread to your body generally before your mastectomy, chemotherapy may be advisable. Ask your physician to review with the pathologist the detailed character of the tumor. Drug treatment may be advisable even if one, two, three, or even five years have elapsed since the date of your mastectomy.

Informed Consent. Much has been written in recent years about informed consent, and much of it makes sense. You must insist that you be fully informed and not given the brush-off. It is by no means easy. It is not just that some doctors resist giving information to their patients, saying, "I am the doctor, leave it to me"; sometimes they really do not know. No doctor knows everything, but the good doctor faced with any problem indicates the limit of his knowledge.

Informed consent is by no means satisfactorily provided by seeking a consultation. Too often the consultant may hold the same opinion as the primary doctor. Here your responsibility for your own health becomes paramount. The better informed you are, the better your questions and the more informative become the answers. Too many breasts are cut off, too many uteruses and ovaries removed, for want of adequate questioning by the woman and understanding on the part of her doctor. If you are not properly informed, you are forced into accepting your doctor's advice and the possibility of a more radical and expensive treatment than is actually needed.

Selecting Your Physician. You are lucky if you have an understanding physician with sufficient time to pay attention to your needs. The list of matters important to your health, as we already know, is a long one, and it won't be easy for any single physician to cover everything himself. He must have the interest and patience to listen to the problems you face, to examine your breasts, your thyroid gland, ovaries, and uterus. If he is to teach you about proper care of yourself, he must have your confidence and a sense of your emotional balance. If your doctor is a member of a group of physicians representing different disciplines, either as an organized clinic or an informal community association, the advice you and the doctor need from neighboring fields can be easily obtained.

Nurse practitioners are now often to be found in such groups. Their contributions are well recognized, and they are being trained in increasing numbers. They can do much in support of the physician. For example, they are as able as he to teach self-examination of the breasts, and they themselves are excellent in examining the breasts, the uterus, and the ovaries.

If the only doctors available are those working alone, it may be more difficult for you to find the appropriate one. Many solo practitioners are often too busy to give the patient more than brief attention, and some are so busy that they are unable to respond. When you meet your physician, tell him your doubts and ask him your questions. If he responds, well and good. If not, seek another. Many gynecologists are today providing general care for their patients. Nurses and social workers know physicians well, and will be able to advise you regarding who are the more approachable doctors.

If your physician demurs about advice regarding your breasts, show him this book. Point out that the notes quote the scientific authorities for each major opinion. Offer to get him a particular article from his hospital's library to save him the trouble, and then ask him to discuss it with you. (You will, of course, have read the article yourself while getting it for him!)

Throughout all these conferences and this growing contact with your physician, you will be expanding your experience and your own responsibility for your health. I cannot overemphasize that good care will depend more on you than on any other factor.

The Woman's Care Center. Young women have so much to learn about themselves in preparation for living and bearing children, if they choose to have children; and older women so much about care of themselves, their children, family, and others, that we at the Massachusetts General Hospital are at the present time setting up a special ambulatory facility, a walk-in clinic. We are aiming to help women deal with their special problems. Already we have learned a lot, with much more still to be realized. We are building more than just a gynecology clinic or obstetrical or breast clinic. The staff consists of surgeon, gynecologist, internist, oncologist, pathologist, psychiatrist, medical student, nurse practitioner, social worker, and secretary, each learning, each contributing. We call it the Woman's Care Center, for the special problems of women.

Human beings become frightened when they are ill, largely because their questions go unanswered, their concerns unrecognized. They are suddenly alone amongst a host of professionals, all of whom are too busy to sit down quietly to explain or give reassurance.

It is my hope that the preceding chapters have given you knowledge, perspective, and confidence. Your care is in your own hands. You should continue to question the way society treats you. Challenge what seems wrong, not stridently, not with anger, but with the gifts and qualities that you possess because you are a woman.

Acknowledgments

FOR WHAT I KNOW of the sciences of medicine I am grateful to my teachers of science in school, college, and medical school; for the technical, surgical care of patients, to my preceptors in the graduate training program when I was a resident surgeon; what I have learned of women's pain and the trials of breast disease I have learned from my patients.

The tutelage in science was systematic, painstaking and accurate. (When an undergraduate I thought of becoming a chemist.) It taught me what was chemically clean. But chemistry was precise and cold; not intriguing, like the vagaries of human beings. And so it was other mentors who dissuaded me by precept, not command, to abandon cold chemistry for human medicine — three lawyers, two musicians, a fisherman port-pilot, a stonemason, a carpenter, a banker, an older doctor whose shaky hands had changed him from surgeon to general practitioner, a determined mother who ruled as a matriarch (my father had died when I was two months old) — all of them individuals who dealt with people, often troubled people. To them I owe most of what is in this book.

The surgical preceptors showed me how an operation could be skillfully done. They trained me in technical proficiency, one of the many necessities of good care of patients. But such training often did not include thought for the patient's deep inner, personal feelings. My respect for such feelings has come for the most part from the patients themselves. They told me their troubles, which in turn led me to question traditional care of breast cancer. I had to look into less disrupting alternative treatments. Without the strength and conviction of the patients nothing would have happened. To these patients my heart-felt thanks.

There are many others to whom I owe much — my wife above all, intimate friends, the several secretaries who have aided me at every turn, and my professional colleagues. I could not have appreciated what the patients were telling me had I not been encouraged by my psychiatrist-friends, particularly Dr. Stanley Cobb and Dr. Grete Bibring. What I have learned about breast cancer I also owe to many; in particular, Benjamin Castleman, William Davies Sohier, and Chiu-an Wang, to mention but three.

There have also been other invaluable experiences. The pursuit of the role of behavioral science in medicine by Professor Jerrold Zacharias, Dr. Douglas Bond, Dr. Bibring, and myself has been supported by the Carnegie Corporation of New York and the Commonwealth Fund. Miss Margaret Mahoney has stimulated new studies into the special care needed by women. To them all I owe much.

And then in the preparation of the manuscript I have been fortunate in benefiting from the skill of Mrs. Ruth Hapgood, who helped me to make this more nearly the book I hoped to write.

How fortunate I have been.

Glossary
Illustrations
Appendix
Notes and Sources
Index

Glossary

Adenofibroma: A benign growth (neoplasm) of both gland cells and fibrous tissue cells.

Adenoma: A benign growth (neoplasm) of gland cells.

Adrenalectomy: Surgical removal of an adrenal gland. (See Bilateral.)

Atom: The smallest particle of an element, which combines with other atoms to form chemical compounds. Atoms are also parts of a molecule.

Atrophy: Decrease in size of an organ, for example, thinning of the skin, decrease in thickness of a muscle, or decrease in size of the breasts after the menopause.

Axilla: Armpit

Bilateral: On both sides. For example, *bilateral adrenalectomy* means removal of both adrenal glands, one on each side of the body; bilateral ovariectomy, removal of both ovaries.

Biopsy: Removal of living cells or a piece of living tissue for diagnostic examination under the microscope.

Carcinoma: A malignant growth (neoplasm) of gland cells, brain cells, cells forming the outer covering-layer of the skin and the mucous membranes of the mouth, throat, stomach, intestines, vagina, and bladder. (Compare Sarcoma.)

Catamenia: Menstruation, from the Greek word *katamenios*, meaning "monthly."

Chemotherapy: Treatment by drugs (chemical treatment).

Cyst: A collection of fluid usually held within a capsule of fibrous tissue or gland cells.

Ductal dysplasia: The greater than normal increase in ductal tissues frequently found as part of the fibrocystic disorder.

Edema: Accumulation of an excess of tissue fluid; a puddling of lymphatic fluid. May be localized in one spot or generalized over the entire body.

Endometrium: The gland-cell lining of the uterus.

Excise: Cut out by sharp surgical instrument, scalpel, or scissors. (See also Resect.)

Excisional biopsy: Removal of an entire lump, or segment of an organ containing a lump, for diagnostic examination under the microscope. (Compare with the more limited, lesser surgical Biopsy.)

Fascia: A thin sheath of connective (fibrous) tissue surrounding muscles and most organs, permitting them to move without dragging the neighboring organs as well.

Fibrocystic disorder: Diffuse proliferation of the fibrous tissue of the breasts, often with formation of cysts. The gland and duct cells may also proliferate as part of the disorder.

Fibroma: A benign growth (neoplasm) of fibrous tissue cells.

Frozen section: For the pathologist to obtain a quick answer regarding possible cancer in an organ, a piece of the organ is removed (a biopsy), is frozen, and a thin slice cut from the frozen block. The slice is then stained and examined under the microscope.

Hematoma: A swelling containing blood, usually the result of a blow. Sometimes the blood becomes confined within a capsule in a well-formed cyst.

Hyperplasia: An increased number of cells, nonmalignant in character, occurring throughout a tissue.

Hypoplasia: A decrease in the number of normal cells. (Compare with Hyperplasia; see also Atrophy.)

Immunotherapy: Treatment by immunization, such as vaccination.

In situ: Literally "in place," *in situ* is used to indicate that germinating cancer cells have remained in the area of origin, that is, they have not invaded outward.

Isotope: One of two or more forms of a single chemical element, one of which may be radioactive, the other(s) not; for example, cobalt and radioactive cobalt; iodine and radioactive iodine.

Lipoma: A benign circumscribed growth of fat cells.

Lumpectomy: The surgical operation of removing a lump.

Lymph: The clear fluid that flows from the tissue spaces to rejoin the blood above the heart. In contrast to blood, lymph normally contains no cells, but cancer cells may float off in it.

Lymph node: A small encapsulated organ of germinating lymph cells. Distributed throughout the body, lymph nodes lie along lymphatic vessels, acting as sieves to catch bacteria and providing lymph cells to the circulation to help fight infection. (The nodes are sometimes mistakenly called lymph glands.)

Lymphatic circulation: The so-called third circulation, it carries the lymph formed in the tissues back to the blood just above the heart.

Lymphatic vessels: The fine, delicate, almost imperceptible vessels that carry the lymph from all tissues of the body back to the general circulation (the blood stream).

Mammogram: A picture of the breast usually taken by passing x-rays throughout the breast and recording the image on x-ray film.

Mastectomy: The surgical operation of removing the breast.

Metastasis: The transfer or spread of cancer from the primary tumor to other areas of the body; for example, to bones, lungs, or liver.

Mitosis: The final process of a cell dividing into two cells. Each new cell takes half of the chromosomes with it. Under the microscope the chromatin material can be seen being pulled apart. At this phase, the cell is called a mitotic figure. The number of such figures is a measure of the rate of growth of a tumor.

Molecule: The smallest particle of an element or chemical compound that is stable; that is, can exist by itself. A molecule is made up of one, two, or more atoms.

Needle aspiration: Insertion of a hollow needle with withdrawal of fluid from a cyst, a hematoma, or other collection of fluid.

Needle biopsy: Removal of cells for examination under the microscope by means of a large needle, with suction applied at outer end of needle.

Neoplasm: A localized growth of abnormal cells. The neoplasm may be either benign or malignant.

Oncology: A specialty of medical knowledge and nonsurgical practice dealing with benign and malignant growths.

Osteoporosis: Thinning of the bones. (Literally, "porous bones.")

Papillary carcinoma: A malignant tumor, the outer surface of which is covered by small nipplelike projections of cells.

Papilloma: A benign, circumscribed growth, the surface of which is covered with small nipplelike projections. (Compare with Papillary carcinoma.)

Peritonitis: Inflammation of the peritoneal (abdominal) cavity, usually by infection.

Perineural invasion: Invasion of nerve sheaths by spreading cancer cells.

Puerperal sepsis: Infection at childbirth; childbirth fever.

Resect: Removal by a sharp surgical instrument, scalpel, or scissors. (See also Excise.)

Sarcoma: A malignant growth (neoplasm) of the supporting tissues of fibrous cell origin. Included are the connective tissue in organs throughout the body, the fibrous tissue of the breast, bones, tendons, and muscles. (Compare Carcinoma.)

Scalpel: A sharp surgical knife with fine point and rounded blade.

Sclerosing adenosis: The greater than normal increase in gland cells, frequently a part of the fibrocystic disorder.

S-phase: The midphase of a cell's preparation to divide. It is the metabolically active phase when the amount of DNA within the cell is doubled and the cell is most vulnerable to drugs.

Surgical biopsy: Removal of a slice of living tissue through an open surgical wound, for examination under the microscope.

Trauma: An injury.

Traumatic: Injurious. A traumatic wound is one produced by violence.

Undifferentiated cell: An immature, childlike, or fetal-like cell. Cancer cells are frequently of such immature character.

Uterine cervix: The neck or outlet of the uterus.

Xeromammogram: A picture of the breast taken by passing x-rays through the breast but recording the image on charged Xerox paper rather than on x-ray film.

Drawings Showing the Lymphatic Drainage from a Cancer in the Breast

Fig. A.
VIEW OF THE RIGHT BREAST FROM THE FRONT

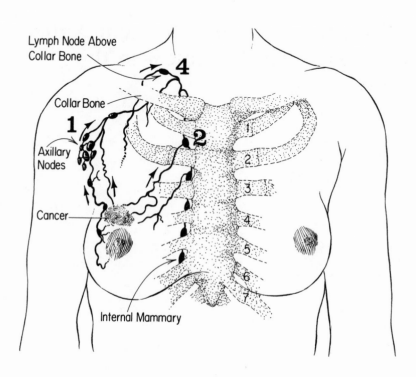

Lymph vessels carry lymph to 4 groups of lymph nodes and from them to the bloodstream at the base of the neck.[1-5] The node groups are: (1) Axillary; (2) Internal mammary, and (4) above the collar bone. The lymph vessels along the ribs leading to the nodes in the back of the chest (group 3) are not visible from in front.

Fig. B.
VIEW OF THE RIGHT BREAST FROM THE RIGHT SIDE, WITH THE CHEST WALL REMOVED EXCEPT FOR THE 5TH RIB

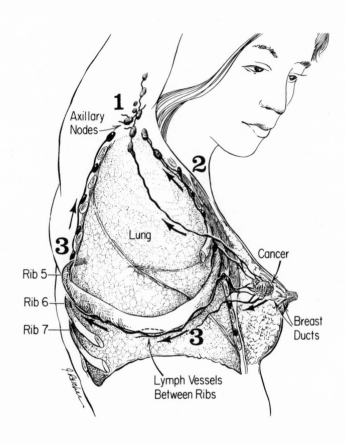

The 3 lobes of the right lung are exposed. The axillary lymph nodes (1) and the lymph vessel to them from the breast are depicted at the base of the uplifted arm. The internal mammary nodes (2) are shown beneath the chest wall in front of the lung. The posterior nodes (3) are illustrated behind the lung between the ribs with the lymph vessel beneath the 5th rib carrying lymph from the breast.[2,4,5] The nodes above the collar bone (4) are not illustrated because they are carried upward out of the picture by the raising of the arm.

COMMENTS

Four operations removing the entire breast are currently used to treat breast cancer. Three of them also resect some of the lymph nodes. None of the 3 removes all of the four groups of nodes which theoretically may harbor cancer cells. The radical mastectomy resects only the group 1 nodes (the axillary); group 2, 3, and 4 nodes are left untouched. The modified radical resects some but not necessarily all of group 1. The superradical removes both group 1 and group 2 nodes. This operation is now seldom recommended. The fourth operation, simple or total mastectomy, removes no nodes.

The American Cancer Society currently recommends the radical or modified radical as the treatment of choice.

The Breast Cancer Task Force of the National Cancer Institute is at present conducting studies to determine which of the three operations, radical, modified radical, or simple, leads to the best result. (The superradical is not included in the study.) Since none of the operations removes more than 50 to 60 percent of the possible nodal involvement, it should not be surprising that the initial results indicate no difference in the outcome whether nodes are included or not.

Primary irradiation hits all four node groups.

Appendix

MATTERS reserved for this appendix are four: breast self-examination, which all women should consider a part of their mature life; remedial measures should they lose a breast; helpful contacts with neighbors should they ever prove to have an incurable cancer; and, fourth, helpful thoughts for them and their families should death become unavoidable.

Breast Self-Examination. The American Cancer Society, the American College of Obstetricians and Gynecologists, and many physicians recommend that all women practice self-examination of their breasts. The pamphlet "Breast Problems in Women," prepared in 1976 by the American College of Obstetricians and Gynecologists, is simple and clear. It is reproduced in part here with the kind permission of the College.

Copies of this pamphlet are available on request to any physician or the American College of Obstetricians and Gynecologists, Suite 2700, One East Wacker Drive, Chicago, Illinois 60601.

Reach To Recovery. Formal psychological support for the woman who undergoes a mastectomy for breast cancer did not come until 1952, when Terese Lasser organized the Reach To Recovery program. She herself had had a mastectomy and, suffering through the consequences, she was determined to help others facing the same problems. Despite indifference on the part of many surgeons, she insisted on being heard. In 1969 the American Cancer Society formally adopted the program.*

The program depends on volunteers, women who have been through a mastectomy and are judged by their physicians to

*Terese Lasser, with the collaboration of William K. Clarke, published a book in 1972, an account of her experiences.

have made a satisfactory emotional adjustment to the loss of their breast. As volunteers they are trained to reassure and encourage women who have just undergone a mastectomy. They visit the patient as early as a day or two after the operation, while she is still in the hospital. They talk with her about what to expect, what to wear over the operative site, where to go to purchase a specially designed substitute brassiere, and generally offer support. The woman's surgeon or physician must ask for this help through the regional local office of the American Cancer Society.

Make Today Count. Patients who have been told they have an incurable disease more often than not feel lost and deserted. Women who have come to realize that their breast cancer is out of control are not exceptions. They need help and support in one form or another. Orville Kelly, a cancer patient from Burlington, Iowa, wrote an article about his worries, and immediately afterward he was deluged with calls from others suffering from comparable troubles. Mr. Kelly conceived of the idea of their meeting together to discuss their problems. "In sharing our problems we discovered that anger, fear, depression, rejection and sexual problems were often more difficult to contend with than cancer." Out of their meetings grew the amazingly helpful organization Make Today Count.

"It is imperative," says Mr. Kelly, "that more than the disease be treated — that the whole person and the family be considered and that, when possible, practical advice be given."*

From the simple beginning, under Mr. Kelly's leadership, a national organization has emerged. By 1976, fifty-four chapters of Make Today Count had been formed across the country. In addition to people with cancer, the chapters include doctors, nurses, and clergymen. Information about the groups can be obtained by writing to Make Today Count, Box 303, Burlington, Iowa 52601.

---

*Medical News, *JAMA (Journal of the American Medical Association)*, 235:2065, 1976.

*On Death and Dying.** Dr. Elisabeth Kübler-Ross, a psychiatrist, has written an extraordinary book about what people go through when they face death from illness. She describes what sick people told her in organized interview seminars she conducted in a Chicago hospital for two and a half years. She also tells how she went about helping them with their worries. The book is about life and all its problems. The reading of it is worthwhile for all of us.

How does one self-examine?

Stand in front of a mirror, arms at your sides. Look for dimpling of the skin of the breast, puckering, or retraction of the nipples, and changes in the breast size or shape. Look for the same signs with your hands pressed tightly on your hips and then with your arms raised high.(1)

Next, lie flat on your back. Place a folded towel under your left shoulder and place your left hand under your head. With

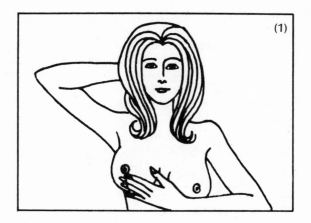

On Death and Dying (New York: Macmillan Co., 1969), 16th printing, 1976.

your right hand, keeping the fingers flat and together, gently feel your left breast using small circular motions with your fingers.(2) Picture your breast as the face of a clock. Begin your small circles at 12 o'clock, then repeat the circular motion at 1 o'clock, and so on.(3) Last, examine the nipple area in the same way. Examine the area below the armpit, which also contains breast tissue and should not be missed. Lower your right arm to your side and reverse the procedure, placing the folded towel under your right shoulder, right hand under your head, and using your left hand to feel your right breast.

When showering or bathing, examination of the skin, smooth and wet with soap and water is also helpful.

Many women have lumpy breasts. The important thing for you to keep in mind is that you are looking for something new or unusual:

— a lump
— thickening or hardening under the skin, discharge
— bleeding
— puckering
— dimpling
— an unusual appearance of the skin or nipple.

If any of these signs are found, alert your physician as soon as possible.

When a physician sees a patient complaining of a change in her breast, he does a complete, meticulous breast examination in pretty much the same manner that the woman has been examining her own breast. He evaluates the risk factors, which include:

— a late menopause
— a history of chronic cystic breast disease
— a history of known premalignant breast lesions
— family history of breast cancer
— previous exposure to high doses of x-ray
— the use of certain drugs and hormones.

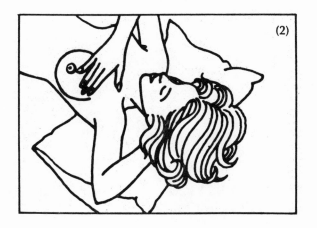

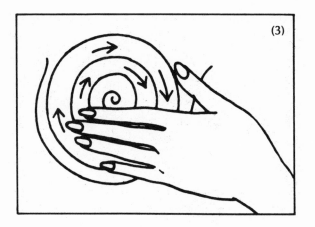

Notes and Sources

Chapter 1
Why This Book? pages 1–4

1. Silverberg, B. S., and Holleb, A. I.: "Major trends in cancer: 25-years survey," *CA: A Cancer Journal for Clinicians*, American Cancer Society, 25:2–21, 1975.
2. Third national cancer survey, incidence data, National Cancer Institute Monograph 41, Cutler, S. J., and Young, J. L., eds., March 1975.
3. Cutler, S. J., and Davesa, S. S. "Trends in cancer incidence and mortality in the U.S.A.," in Doll, R., and Vodopija, I. *Host Environment Interactions in the Etiology of Cancer in Man* (Lyon: International Agency for Research on Cancer, 1970.)

Chapter 2
Four Women pages 5–15

1. "American Cancer Society's Policy Statement on the Surgical Treatment of Breast Cancer: Current official position of the American Cancer Society," *Cancer*, 23:341, 1975.
2. Fisher, B., Wolmark, N. "New concepts in the management of primary breast cancer," *Cancer*, 36:627–632, 1975.
3. Nathanson, I. T., Kelley, R. M., "Hormonal treatment of cancer," *New Eng. J. Med.*, 246:135, 1952.
4. Cope, O., Wang, C. A., Chu, A., et al. "Limited surgical excision as the basis of a comprehensive therapy for cancer of the breast," *Am. J. Surg.*, 131:400–407, 1976.
5. Huggins, C., Dao, T.L. "Adrenalectomy for mammary cancer," *Ann. Surg.*, 136:595–603, 1950.

Chapter 3
The Biology of the Normal Breast and Its Everyday Troubles pages 16–26

1. Linzell, J. L., and Peaker, M. "Mechanism of milk secretion," *Physiol. Rev.*, 51:564–596, 1971.

2. Jones, C. H., Greening, W. P., Davey, J. B., et al. "Thermography aids breast cancer search," *Br. J. Radiol.*, 48:532–538, 1975.

3. Ezrin, C. "Introduction to endocrinology," Chapter 1, in *Systematic Endocrinology*, Ezrin, C., Godden, J. O., Volpe, R., and Wilson, R., eds. (New York: Harper & Row, 1973).

4. Leis, H. P. "Hormones in the epidemiology of breast cancer," *Breast: Diseases of the Breast*, 2:7–13, 1976.

5. Mittra, I., and Hayward, J. L. "Hypothalamic-pituitary-prolactin axis in breast cancer," *Lancet*, 1:889–891, 1974.

6. Nathanson, I. T. "Present concepts of benign breast disease," *N. Eng. J. Med.*, 235:516–520, 548–563, 1946.

7. Frantz, V. K., Pickren, J. W., Melcher, G. W., et al. "Incidence of chronic cystic disease in so-called 'normal breasts:' a study based on 225 postmortem examinations," *Cancer*, 4:762–782, 1951.

8. Ackerman, L. V., and Rosai, J. "Breast," Chapter 19 in *Surgical Pathology*, 5th ed. (St. Louis: C. V. Mosby Co., 1974).

Chapter 4

Breast Tumors, Benign and Malignant   pages 27–37

1. Ackerman, L. V., and Rosai, J. "Breast," Chapter 19 in *Surgical Pathology*, 5th ed. (St. Louis: C. V. Mosby Co., 1974).

2. Ackerman, L. V., and Rosai, J. "The pathology of tumors," Part Four, "Grading, staging and classification of neoplasms," *CA: A Cancer Journal for Clinicians*, American Cancer Society, 21:368–372, 1971.

3. Fenig, J., Arlen, M., Livingston, S. F., and Levowitz, B. S. "The potential for carcinoma existing synchronously on a microscopic level within the second breast," *Surg., Gynecol., Obstet.*, 141:394–396, 1975.

4. Vickery A. L., Jr. "Case records of the Massachusetts General Hospital. Case 2–1977," *N. Eng. J. Med.*, 296:94–100, 1977.

5. Camp, E. "Inflammatory carcinoma of the breast," *Am. J. Surg.*, 131:583–586, 1976.

6. Blumenson, L. E., and Bross, D. J. "A mathematical analysis of the growth and spread of breast cancer," *Biometrics*, 25:95–109, 1969.

7. Nissen-Meyer, R., Kjellgren, K., and Mansson, B. "Preliminary report from the Scandinavian adjuvant chemotherapy study group," *Cancer Chemother. Rep.*, 55:561–566, 1971.

8. Slack, N. H., Blumenson, L. E., and Bross, I. D. J. "Therapeutic implications from a mathematical model characterizing the course of breast cancer," *Cancer*, 24:960–971, 1969.

9. Friedell, G. H., Betts, A., and Sommers, S. C. "The prognostic value of blood vessel invasion and lymphocytic infiltrates in breast carcinoma," *Cancer*, 18:164–166, 1965.

10. Ruiz, U., Babeu, S., Schwartz, M. S., et al. "Blood vessel invasion and lymph node metastasis: two factors affecting survival in breast cancer," *Surgery*, 73:185–190, 1973.
11. Hoover, R., Mason, T. J., McKay, F. W., et al. "Cancer by county: new resources for etiologic clues," *Science*, 189:1005–1007, 1975.
12. Shapley, D. "Nitrosamines: scientists on the trail of prime suspect in urban cancer," *Science*, 191:268–270, 1976.
13. Braverman, L. E. "Consequences of thyroid radiation in children," *N. Eng. J. Med.*, editorial, 292:204–205, 1975.
14. McKenzie, I. "Breast carcinoma following multiple fluoroscopies," *Br. J. Cancer*, 19:1–8, 1965.
15. deWaard, F. "Diet and nutrition as environmental factors in the pathogenesis of breast cancer," in Report to the Profession: Breast Cancer, National Cancer Institute, September 1974.
16. Bittner, J. J. "Possible relationship of the estrogenic hormones, genetic susceptibility, and milk influence in the production of mammary cancer in mice," *Cancer Res.*, 2:710, 1942.
17. Borden, E. C. "Viruses and breast cancer: Implications of mouse and human studies," *The Johns Hopkins Medical Journal*, 134:66–76, 1974.
18. Kirschner, M. "Relation of endocrine functions to epidemiological characteristics in breast cancer," in Report to the Profession: Breast Cancer, National Cancer Institute, September 1974.
19. Frantz, E. G., Kleinberg, D. L., and Noel, G. L. "Studies on prolactin in man," in *Recent Progress in Hormone Research*, Astwood, E. B., ed. (New York: Academic Press, 1972), 28:527–571.
20. Maloof, F. "Regulatory mechanisms of the pituitary-thyroid axis," Chapter 15, in *Pathophysiology, Altered Regulatory Mechanisms in Disease*, Frohlich, E. D., ed. (Philadelphia: J. B. Lippincott, 1972).
21. Lynch, H. T., Guirgis, H. A., Brodkey, F., et al. "Genetic heterogeneity and familial carcinoma of the breast," *Surg., Gynecol., Obstet.*, 142:693–699, 1976.
22. Crile, G., Jr. "A study of metastases from involved lymph nodes after removal of primary tumors with special reference to cancers of the breast," *Trans. Southern Surgical Association*, 76:131–135, 1964.

Chapter 5

Who Gets Cancer of the Breast   pages 38–51

1. Silverberg, B. S., and Holleb, A. I. "Major trends in cancer: 25-year survey," *CA: A Cancer Journal for Clinicians*, American Cancer Society, 25:2–21, 1975.
2. Third national cancer survey, incidence data, National Cancer In-

stitute Monograph 41, Cutler, S. J. and Young, J. L., eds., March 1975.

3. Cutler, S. J., and Davesa, S. S. "Trends in cancer incidence and mortality in the U.S.A.," in Doll, R., and Vodopija, I. *Host Environment Interactions in the Etiology of Cancer in Man* (Lyon: International Agency for Research on Cancer, 1970).

4. Shimkin, M. B. "Cancer of the breast: Some old facts and new prospectives, *JAMA*, 183:146–149, 1963.

5. Leis, H. P., Jr. "Hormones in the epidemiology of breast cancer," *Breast: Diseases of the Breast*, 2:7–13, 1976.

6. Strax, P. *Early Detection: Breast Cancer Is Curable* (New York: Harper & Row, 1975).

7. Johnson, G. T. *What You Should Know About Health Care Before You Call a Physician*! (New York: McGraw-Hill Book Co., 1975), p. 397.

8. MacMahon, B., Cole, P., and Brown, J. "Etiology of human breast cancer: a review," *J. Natl. Cancer Inst.* 50:21–42, 1973.

9. Broca, P. P. *Traité des tumeurs* (Paris: Asselin, 1866).

10. Lynch, H. T., Krush, A. J., Lemon, H. M., et al. "Tumor variation in families with breast cancer," *JAMA*, 222:1631–1635, 1972.

11. Lynch, H. T., Guirgis, H. A., Brodkey, F., et al. "Genetic heterogeneity and familial carcinoma of the breast," *Surg., Gynecol., Obstet.*, 142:693–699, 1976.

12. Anderson, D. E. "Familial susceptibility to cancer," *CA: A Cancer Journal for Clinicians*, American Cancer Society, 3:143–149, 1976.

13. Hoover, R., Gray, L. A., Sr., Cole, P., et al. "Menopausal estrogens and breast cancer," *N. Eng. J. Med.*, 295:401–405, 1976.

14. Ryan, K. J. "Cancer risk and estrogen use in the menopause," *N. Eng. J. Med.*, editorial, 293:1199–1202.

15. Weiss, N. S. "Risks and benefits of estrogen use," *N. Eng. J. Med.*, editorial, 233:1200–1202, 1975.

16. Marx, J. L. "Estrogen drugs: do they increase the risk of cancer?" *Science*, 191:838–841, 1976.

17. Weiss, N. S., Szekely, D. R., and Austin, D. F. "Increasing incidence of endometrial cancer in the United States," *N. Engl. J. Med.*, 294:1259–1262, 1976.

18. Mack, T. M., Pike, M. C., Henderson, B. E., et al. "Estrogens and endometrial cancer in a retirement community," *N. Eng. J. Med.*, 294:1262–1267, 1976.

19. Manber, M. M. "Diethylstilbestrol," *Medical World News*, August 23, 1976.

20. Sartwell, P. E., Arthes, F. G., and Tonascia, J. A. "Epidemiology of benign breast lesions: lack of association with oral contraceptive use," *N. Eng. J. Med.*, 288:551–554, 1973.

21. Ory, H., Cole, P., MacMahon, B., et al. "Oral contraceptives and

reduced risk of benign breast diseases," *N. Eng. J. Med.*, 294:419–422, 1976.

22. Nathanson, I. T. "Present concepts of benign breast disease," *N. Eng. J. Med.*, 235:516–520, 548–563, 1946.

23. Davis, H. H., Simons, M., and Davis, J. B. "Cystic disease of the breast: relationship to carcinoma," *Cancer*, 17:957–978, 1964.

24. Frantz, V. K., Pickren, J. W., Melcher, G. W., et al. "Incidence of chronic cystic disease in so-called 'normal breasts,' a study based on 225 postmortem examinations," *Cancer*, 4:762–782, 1951.

25. Edelstyn, G. A., Lyons, A. R., and Welbourn, R. B. "Thyroid function in patients with mammary cancer," *Lancet*, 1:670–671, 1958.

26. Bogardus, G. M., and Finley, J. W. "Breast cancer and thyroid disease," *Surgery*, 49:461, 1961.

27. Blackwinkel, K., and Jackson, A. S. "Some features of breast cancer and thyroid deficiency, report of 280 cases," *Cancer* 17:1174–1176, 1964.

28. Mittra, I., and Hayward, J. H. "Hypothalamic-pituitary-thyroid axis in breast cancer," *Lancet*, 1:885–888, 1974.

29. Sadowsky, N. L., Kalisher, L., White, G., et al. "Radiologic detection of breast cancer: review and recommendations," *N. Eng. J. Med.*, 294:370–373, 1976.

30. Unsigned. Medical News, "Critics, defenders express views about routine mammography," *JAMA*, 236:541–542, 1976.

31. Culliton, B. J. "Breast cancer: second thoughts about routine mammography," *Science*, 193:555–558, 1976.

32. Cole, P. "Epidemiology of breast cancer: an overview," in Report to the Profession: Breast Cancer, National Cancer Institute, pp. 11–20, September 1974.

33. Phillips, R. L., "Role of life-style and dietary habits in risk of cancer among Seventh-Day Adventists," *Cancer Res.* 35:13–22, 1975.

34. Lyon, J. L., Klauber, M. R., Gardner, J. W., et al. "Cancer incidence in Mormons and non-Mormons in Utah, 1966-1970," *N. Eng. J. Med.*, 294:129–133, 1976.

Chapter 6
Surgery — The First Hope   pages 52–75

1. Bowditch, N. I. *A history of the Massachusetts General Hospital, 1811 to 1851* (Boston: John Wilson & Son, 1851).

2. Cheyne, Sir W. W. *"Lister and His Achievement: Being the First Lister Memorial Lecture delivered at the Royal College of Surgeons of England on May 14, 1925.* (London: Longmans, Green and Co., 1925).

3. Holleb, A. I. "American Cancer Society policy statement on surgi-

cal treatment of breast cancer," *CA: A Cancer Journal for Clinicians*, 23:341–343, 1975.

4. Halsted, W. S. "The results of operations for the cure of cancer of the breast performed at the Johns Hopkins Hospital from June 1889 to January 1894," *Ann. Surg.*, 20:497–555, 1894.

5. Volkmann, R. von. See reference 4, above.

6. Meyer, W. "Operative technique for cancer of the breast," *Ann. Surg.*, 25:478–480, 1897.

7. Billroth, A. Krankheiten der weiblichen brustdrüse," *Handbuch der Chirurgie*, Billroth and Lücke (Stuttgart: F. Enke, 1880).

8. Halsted, W. S. "A clinical and histological study of certain adenocarcinomata of the breast," *Ann. Surg.*, 28:557–576, 1898.

9. Halsted, W. S. "The results of radical operations for the cure of carcinoma of the breast," *Ann. Surg.*, 46:1–19, 1907.

10. Halsted, W. S. "Developments in the skin-grafting operation for cancer of the breast," *JAMA*, 1x:416–418, 1913.

11. Handley, S. *Cancer of the breast* (London: John Murray, 1906).

12. Urban, J. A. "Clinical experience and results of excision of the internal mammary lymph node chain in primary operable breast cancer," *Cancer*, 12:14–22, 1959.

13. Dahl-Iversen, E., and Tobiassen, T. "Radical mastectomy with parasternal and supraclavicular dissection for mammary carcinoma," *Ann. Surg.*, 170:889–891, 1969.

14. Keynes, G. "The treatment of primary carcinoma of the breast with radium," *Acta Radiol.*, Stockholm, 10:393–401, 1929.

15. Keynes, G. "The place of radium in the treatment of cancer of the breast," *Ann. Surg.*, 106:619–630, 1937.

16. McKittrick, L. S. "Interstitial radiation of cancer of the breast: a review of ninety-six cases of cancer of the breast treated according to the technique of Geoffrey Keynes," *Ann. Surg.*, 106:631–644, 1937.

17. Ross, J. P. "An investigation into the effects of radium upon carcinoma of the breast," *Brit. J. Surg.*, 27:211–223, 1939.

18. McWhirter, R. "Value of simple mastectomy and radiotherapy in the treatment of cancer of the breast," *Brit. J. Radiol.*, 21:599–610, 1948.

19. Patey, D. H., and Dyson, W. H. "The prognosis of carcinoma of the breast in relation to the type of operation performed," *Brit. J. Cancer*, 2:7–13, 1948.

20. Auchincloss, H., Jr. "Significance of location and number of axillary metastases in carcinoma of the breast; a justification for a conservative operation," *Ann. Surg.*, 158:37–46, 1963.

21. Fisher, B., and Wolmark, N. "New concepts in the management of primary breast cancer," *Cancer*, 36:627–632, 1975.

22. Longcope, W. Personal communication, 1937.
23. Olch, P. D. "William S. Halsted and local anesthesia: contributions and complications," *Anaesthesiology*, 42:479–486, 1975.
24. Cope, O. "Breast Cancer: has the time come for a less mutilating treatment?" *Radcliffe Quarterly*, p. 6, June 1970.
25. Cope, O. "Breast cancer: has the time come for a less mutilating treatment?" *Psychiatry Med.*, 2:263–269, 1971.
26. Handley, R. S., and Thackray, A. C. "Conservative radical mastectomy (Patey's operation)," *Ann Surg.*, 170:880–882, 1969.
27. Daland, E. M. "Untreated cancer of the breast," *Surg., Gynecol., and Obstet.*, 44:264–268, 1927.
28. Nathanson, I. T., and Welch, C. E. "Life expectancy and incidence of malignant disease. I. Carcinoma of the breast," *Am. J. Cancer*, 28:40–53, 1936.
29. Harrington, S. W. "Fifteen-year to forty-year survival rates following radical mastectomy for cancer of the breast," *Ann. Surg.*, 137:843–849, 1953.
30. Williams, I. G., Murley, R. S., and Curwen, M. P. "Carcinoma of the female breast: conservative and radical surgery," *Brit. Med. J.*, pp. 787–796, 1953.
31. Berg, J. W., and Robbins, G. F. "Factors influencing short and long term survival of breast cancer patients," *Surg., Gynecol., and Obstet.*, 122:1311–1316, 1966.
32. McLaughlin, C. W., and Coe, J. D. "Cancer of the breast — a continuing challenge: report of 375 consecutive patients with long-term follow-up," *Ann. Surg.*, 169:844–850, 1969.
33. Peters, M. V. "Wedge resection and irradiation: an effective treatment of early breast cancer," *JAMA*, 200:144, 1967.
34. Cutler, S. J., and Heise, H. W. "Long-term end results of treatment of cancer," *JAMA*, 216:293–297, 1971.
35. Lee, R. O., and Lambley, D. G. "Radical mastectomy in the treatment of breast cancer," *Brit. J. Surg.*, 58:137–144, 1971.
36. Campos, J. L. "Observations on the mortality from carcinoma of the breast," *Brit. J. Radiol.*, 45:31–38, 1972.
37. Ruiz, U., Babeu, S., Schwartz, M. S., et al. "Blood vessel invasion and lymph node metastasis: two factors affecting survival in breast cancer," *Surgery*, 73:185–190, 1973.

In addition to the above seven reports, notes 31–37, Dr. J. C. Paymaster and his surgical colleagues at the Tata Memorial Center, Bombay, India, have found the same disappointing results of radical mastectomy in 1200 women operated on from 1941 to 1951 and followed for twenty-five years (Paymaster, J. C., personal communication).

38. Bruce, J. "Operable cancer of the breast: a controlled clinical trial," *Cancer*, 28:1443–1452, 1971.
39. Mustakallio, S. "Conservative treatment of breast carcinoma — review of 25 years follow-up," *Clin. Radiol.*, 23:110–116, 1972.

Chapter 7
Radiation   pages 76–90

1. Roentgen, W. K. "Uber eine neue art von strahlen," *Ann. der Phys.*, 64, 1898.
2. Duane, W. "The scientific basis of short wave-length therapy," *Am. J. Roentgenol.*, 9:781–791, 1922.
3. Trump, J. G., Van de Graaff, R. J., and Cloud, R. W. "Compact supervoltage roentgen ray generator using pressure insulated electrostatic high voltage source," *Am. J. Roentgenol. and Rad. Ther.*, 44:610, 1940.
4. Robbins, L. L., Aub, J. C., Cope, O., et al. "Superficial 'burns' of skin and eyes from scattered cathode rays," *Radiology*, 46:1–23, 1946.
5. Lawrence, E. O. "The medical cyclotron of the William H. Crocker radiation laboratory," *Science*, 90:407–408, 1937.
6. Hertz, S., Roberts, A., Means, J. G., and Evans, R. D. "Radioactive iodine as indicator of thyroid physiology," *Am. J. Physiol.*, 28:565–576, 1940.
7. Schulz, M. D. "The supervoltage story," Janeway Lecture, 1974, *Am. J. Roentgenol. Radium Ther. and Nucl. Med.*, 124:541–559, 1975.
8. Griscom, N. T., and Wang, C. C. "Radiation therapy of inoperable breast carcinoma," *Radiology*, 79:18–23, 1962.
9. Wang, C. C., and Griscom, N. T. "Inflammatory carcinoma of the breast: Results following orthovoltage and supervoltage radiation therapy," *Clin. Radiol.*, 15:168–174, 1964.
10. Hammond, A. "Cancer radiation therapy: potential for high energy particles," *Science*, 175:1230–1232, 1972.
11. Sinclair, W. K. "Cyclic x-ray responses in mammalian cells in vitro," *Rad. Res.*, 33:620–643, 1968.
12. Belli, J. A., and Hellman, S. "Hypoxic cell radiosensitizers," *N. Eng. J. Med.*, 294:1399–1400, 1976.
13. Hall, E. J., Roizin-Towle, L., and Attix, F. "Radiobiological studies with cyclotron-produced neutrons currently used for radiotherapy," *Int. J. Radiat. Oncol. Biol. Phys.* 1:33–41, 1975.
14. Handley, R. S., and Thackray, A. C. "Invasion of the internal mammary lymph glands in carcinoma of the breast," *Br. J. Cancer*, 1:15–20, 1947.

15. Turner-Warwick, R. T. "The lymphatics of the breast," *Br. J. Surg.*, 46:574–582, 1959.

16. Delclos, L., and Montague, E. D. "Metastasis from breast cancer," Chapter 6, *Management of Localized Breast Cancer: Textbook of Radiotherapy*, 2nd ed., Fletcher, G. H., ed. (Philadelphia: Lea & Febiger, 1973).

17. Keynes, G. "The treatment of primary carcinoma of the breast with radium," *Acta Radiol.*, 10:393–401, 1929.

18. McKittrick, L. S. "Interstitial radiation of cancer of the breast," *Ann. Surg.*, 631–644, 1937.

19. Robbins, G. F., Lucas, J. C., Fracchia, A. S., et al. "An evaluation of postoperative prophylactic radiation therapy in breast cancer," *Surg., Gynecol., and Obstet.*, 122:979–982, 1966.

20. Mustakallio, S. "Treatment of breast cancer by tumor extirpation and roentgen therapy instead of radical operation," *J. Faculty of Radiologists*, 6:23–26, 1954.

21. Baclesse F., Ennuyer, A., and Cheguillaune, J. "Est-on autorise a practiquer une tumorectomie simple suivie de radiotherapie en cas de tumeur mammaire?" *J. de Radiologie*, 41:137, 1960.

22. DeWinter, J. G. "Early breast cancer treated by biopsy-excision and therapy: A preliminary report," *IX International Congress of Radiology* 1:781, 1961.

23. Porritt, A. "Early carcinoma of the breast," *Brit. J. Surg.*, 51:214, 1964.

24. Wise, L., Mason, A. Y., and Ackerman, L. V. "Local excision and irradiation: an alternative method for the treatment of early mammary cancer," *Ann. Surg.*, 174:392, 1971.

25. Peters, M. Vera. "Radiation therapy in the management of breast cancer," *Proc. Sixth National Cancer Conference*, Denver, Colorado, Sept. 18–20, 1968.

26. Mustakallio, S. "Conservative treatment of breast carcinoma — review of 25 years follow-up," *Clin. Radiol.*, 23:110, 1972.

27. Rissanen, P. M., and Holsti, P. "Vergleich zwischen konservativer und radikaler chirurgie, komginiert mit Strahlentherapie, bei der Behandlung des Brustkrebses im Stadium I," *Strahlentherapie*, 147:370–374, 1974.

28. Guttman, R. J. "Survival and results after 2-million volt irradiation in the treatment of primary operable carcinoma of the breast with proved positive internal mammary and/or highest axillary nodes," *Cancer*, 15:383–386, 1962.

29. Guttman, R. J. "Radiotherapy in the treatment of primary operable carcinoma of the breast with proved lymph node metastases," *Am. J. Roentgenol. Radium Ther. and Nucl. Med.*, 89:58–63, 1963.

30. Nelson, A. J. III, and Montague, E. D. "Resectable localized breast cancer," *JAMA*, 231:189–191, 1975.

31. Prosnitz, L. R., and Goldenberg, I. S. "Irradiation for early breast Ca.," *Medical World News*, p. 31, February 1975.

32. Webber, E., and Hellman, S. "Radiation as primary treatment for local control of breast carcinoma — a progress report," *JAMA*, 243:608–611, 1975.

33. McWhirter, R. "Value of simple mastectomy and radiotherapy in the treatment of cancer of the breast," *Brit. J. Radiol.*, 21:599–610, 1948.

34. Bruce, J. "Operable cancer of the breast; a controlled clinical trial," *Cancer*, 28:1443–1452, 1971.

35. Cope, O., Wang, C. A., Schulz, M., et al. "Breast cancer reconsidered: the rationale for radiation therapy without mastectomy," *Trans. The New England Surgical Society*, October 1967.

36. Cope, O., Wang, C. A., Chu, A., et al. "Limited surgical excision as the basis of a comprehensive therapy for cancer of the breast," *Am. J. Surg.*, 131:400–407, 1976.

37. Moore, G. In discussion of Fisher, B., Slack, N. H., and Cavanaugh, P. J. "Postoperative radiotherapy in the treatment of breast cancer: results of the NSABP clinical trial," *Ann. Surg.*, 172:711, 1972.

38. Humphrey, J. J., and Hammond, W. G. "Treatment of primary breast cancer: change without improvement," *Arch. Surg.*, 104:260, 1972.

39. Forrest, A. P. M. "Discussion of breast cancer therapy: reports of the spring meeting, American College of Surgeons," *Surg. Congress News*, 2:1, 1974.

40. Handley, R. S. "A surgeon's view of the spread of breast cancer," *Cancer*, 24:1231, 1969.

41. Bross, I. D. J. "Scientific strategies in human affairs: use of deep mathematical models," *Trans. N.Y. Acad. Sci.* (Series 11) 34:187, 1972.

42. Cooper, R. G. "Combination chemotherapy in hormone resistant breast cancer," *Proc. Am. Assoc. Cancer Res.*, 10:15, 1969.

43. Zubrod, C. G. "The basis for progress in chemotherapy," *Cancer*, 30:1474, 1972.

44. Kelley, R. M. "What chemotherapy should be used in metastatic breast cancer?" p. 137, *Recent Results in Cancer Research*, Vol. 42, Griem, M. L., Jense, E. V., Ultmann, J. E., and Wissler, R. W., eds. (New York: Springer-Verlag, 1973).

45. Kaufman, S. "Disseminated carcinoma of the breast: principles of treatment," *Geriatrics*, 28:135, 1973.

46. Ackerman, L. V., and Rosai, J. "The pathology of tumors, Part Four: grading, staging and classification of neoplasms," *CA: A Cancer Journal for Clinicians*, 21:368, 1971.

Chapter 8
Hormone Therapy   pages 91–99

1. Beatson, G. T. "On the treatment of inoperable cases of carcinoma of the mamma: suggestions for a new method of treatment with illustrative cases," *Lancet*, 2:104–107, 162–165, 1896.
2. McMahon, C. E., and Cahill, J. L. "The evolution of the concept of the use of surgical castration and in the palliation of breast cancer in premenopausal females," *Ann. Surg.*, 184:713–716, 1976.
3. Boyd, S. "On oophorectomy in cancer of breast," *Br. Med. J.*, 2:1161, 1900.
4. Taylor, G. W. "Evaluation of ovarian sterilization for breast cancer," *Surg., Gynec., and Obstet.*, 68:452–456, 1939.
5. Nathanson, I. T., and Kelley, R. M. "Hormonal treatment of cancer," *N. Eng. J. Med.*, 246:135, 1952.
6. Fracchia, A. A., Murray, D. R., Farrow, J. H., et al. "Comparison of prophylactic and therapeutic castration in breast carcinoma," *Surg., Gynecol., and Obstet.*, 129:270–276, 1969.
7. O'Bryan, R. M., Gordan, G. S., Kelley, R. M., et al. "Does thyroid substance improve response of breast cancer to surgical castration?" *Cancer*, 33:1082–1085, 1974.
8. Veronesi, U., Pizzocaro, G., and Rossi, A. "Oophorectomy for advanced carcinoma of the breast," *Surg., Gynec., and Obstet.*, 141:569, 1975.
9. White, J. W. "The present position of the surgery of the hypertrophied prostate," *Ann. Surg.*, 18:152–188, 1893.
10. Cabot, A. T. "The question of castration for enlarged prostate," *Ann. Surg.*, 24:265–285, 1896.
11. Young, H. H. *Modern urology*, Cabot, H., ed. (Philadelphia: Lea & Febiger, 1936), 1:713.
12. Maloof, F. Personal communication.
13. Mittra, I., and Hayward, J. L. "Hypothalamic-pituitary-thyroid axis in breast cancer," *Lancet*, 1:885–888, 1974.
14. Loeser, A. A. "A new therapy for prevention of post-operative recurrences in genital and breast cancer: a six-year study of prophylactic thyroid treatment," *Br. Med. J.*, 2:1380–1383, 1954.
15. Masnick, G. "Regular breastfeeding can result in contraception, sociologist reports," *Harvard University Gazette*, 9 April 1976, pp. 3 and 7.

16. McCracken, J. A. "Prostaglandins and luteal regression," in *Research in Prostaglandins*, publication of the Prostaglandin Information Center of the Worcester Foundation, 1:1–4, 1972.
17. Kolata, G. B. L. "Thromboxanes: the power behind the prostaglandins?" *Science*, 190:770–771, 812, 1975.
18. Seyberth, H. W., Segre, G. V., Morgan, J. L., et al. "Prostaglandins as mediators of hypercalcemia associated with certain types of cancer." *N. Eng. J. Med.*, 293:1278–1282, 1975.
19. Locke, W., and Schally, A. V. *The Hypothalamus and Pituitary in Health and Disease* (Springfield, Ill.: Charles C. Thomas, 1972), and Segaloff, A. "Hormone treatment of breast cancer," *JAMA*, 1175–1177, 1975.
20. Richardson, E. P., Aub, J. C., and Bauer, W. "Parathyroidectomy in osteomalacia," *Ann. Surg.*, 90:730–741, 1929.
21. Bauer, W., Albright, F., and Aub, J. C. "A case of osteitis fibrosa cystica (osteomalacia?) with evidence of hyperactivity of the parathyroid bodies," Metabolic Study II., *J. Clin. Invest.*, 8:229–248, 1930.
22. Bauer, W., and Aub, J. C. "Studies of calcium and phosphorus metabolism, XVI: the influence of the pituitary gland," *J. Clin. Invest.*, 20:295–301, 1941.
23. Nathanson, I. T., and Aub, J. C. "Excretion of sex hormones in abnormalities of puberty," *J. Clin. Endocrinol.*, 3:321–330, 1943.
24. Lacassagne, A. "Apparition d'adenocarcinomes mammaires chez des souris males traitées par une substance oestrogene synthetique." *C. R. Soc. Biol.* (Paris), 129:641, 1932.
25. Nathanson, I. T. "Hormonal alteration of advanced cancer of the breast," *Surg. Clin. North Am.*, 1144–1150, 1947.
26. Huggins, C., and Scott, W. W. "Bilateral adrenalectomy in prostatic cancer," *Ann. Surg.*, 122:1031–1041, 1945.
27. Huggins, C., and Dao, T. L. "Adrenalectomy for mammary cancer," *Ann. Surg.*, 136:595–603, 1950.
28. Sohier, W. D., and Kelley, R. M. Personal communication.
29. Lemon, H. M. "Prednisone therapy of advanced mammary cancer," *Cancer*, 12:93–107, 1959.
30. Stoll, B. A. "Corticosteriods in therapy of advanced mammary cancer," *Br. Med. J.*, 2:210–214, 1963.
31. Santen, R. J., Lipton, A., and Kendall, J. "Successful medical adrenalectomy with amino-glutethimide," *JAMA*, 230:1661–1665, 1974.
32. Pearson, O. H., and Ray, B. S. "Results of hypophysectomy in the treatment of metastatic mammary carcinoma," *Cancer*, 12:85–92, 1959.

33. Luft, R., and Olivecrona, H. "Experiences with hypophysectomy in man," *J. Neurosurg.*, 10:301–316, 1953.
34. Macdonald, I. "Adrenalectomy and hypophysectomy in disseminated mammary carcinoma: a preliminary statement by the Joint Committee on Endocrine Ablative Procedures in Disseminated Mammary Carcinoma," *JAMA*, 175:787–790, 1961.
35. Atkins, H., Falconer, M. A., Hayward, J. L., et al. "The timing of adrenalectomy and of hypophysectomy in the treatment of advanced breast cancer," *Lancet*, 1:827–830, 1966.
36. McGuire, W. L. "Estrogen receptors in human breast cancer," *J. Clin. Invest.*, 52:73–77, 1973.
37. Horwitz, K. D., and McGuire, W. L. "Predicting response to endocrine therapy in human breast cancer: a hypothesis," *Science*, 189:726–727, 1975.
38. Singhakowinta, A., Potter, H. G., Buroker, D. O., et al. "Estrogen receptor and natural course of breast cancer," *Ann. Surg.*, 183:84–88, 1976.
39. Sasaki, G. H., Leung, B. S., and Fletcher, W. S. "LevoDopa test and estrogen receptor assay in prognosticating responses of patients with advanced cancer of the breast to endocrine therapy," *Ann. Surg.*, 183:392–396, 1976.

Chapter 9

Chemotherapy — The New Hope   pages 100–126

1. Dale, H. H. Preface in *Collected Papers*, Vol. II, *Immunology and Cancer Research*, Himmelweit, F., ed. (London: Pergamon Press, 1957), p. 55.
2. Koch, R. "On bacteriology and its results," lecture delivered at First General Meeting of Tenth International Medical Conference, Berlin, trans. by T. W. Hime (London: Bailliere, Tindall & Cox, 1890).
3. Beveridge, W. I. B. *The Art of Scientific Investigation*, revised ed. (New York: W. W. Norton & Co., Inc., 1957).
4. Ehrlich, P. *Collected Papers of*, Vol. II, *Immunology and Cancer Research*, Himmelweit, F., ed. (London: Pergamon Press, 1957), pp. 235–239.
5. Goodman, L. S., and Gilman, A. *The Pharmacological Basis of Therapeutics*, 4th ed. (London: Collier-Macmillan Ltd., 1970), p. 174.
6. Domagk, G. "Ein beitrag zur chemotherapie der bakteriellen infektionen," *Dt. med. Wschr.*, 61:250–253, 1935a.
7. Tréfouël, J., Tréfouël, Mme. J., Nitti, F., and Bovet, D. "Activité

du p-aminophenysulfamide sur les infections streptococciques experimentales de la souris et du lapin," *C. r. Séanc. Soc. Biol.*, 120:756–758, 1935.

8. Colebrook, L., and Kenny, M. "Treatment of human puerperal infections, and of experimental infections in mice, with Prontosil," *Lancet*, 1:1279–1286, 1936.

9. Long, P. H., and Bliss, E. A. "Para-amino-benzenesulfonamide and its derivatives, experimental and clinical observations on their use in treatment of beta hemolytic streptococci infection: preliminary report," *JAMA*, 108:32–37, 1937.

10. Haddow, A. "The influence of carcinogenic substances on sarcoma induced by the same and other compounds," *J. Pathol.*, 47:581–591, 1938.

11. Fleming, A. "On the antibacterial action of cultures of a pencillium with special reference to their use in the isolation of B. influenzae," *Brit. J. Exper. Pathol.*, 10:226–236, 1929.

12. Florey, H. W., Chain, E., Heatley, N. G., et al. "Penicillin as a chemotherapeutic agent," *Lancet*, 2:226–228, 1940.

13. Dubos, R. J. "Effect of specific agents extracted from soil microorganisms upon experimental bacterial infections," *Ann. Int. Med.*, 13:2025–2037, 1940.

14. Waksman, S. A., Bugie, E., and Schatz, A. "Isolation of antibiotic substances from soil micro-organisms with special reference to streptothricin and streptomycin," Mayo Foundation Lecture, *Proc. Staff Mtg., Mayo Clinic*, 19:537–548, 1944.

15. Gilman, A., and Philips, F. S. "The biological actions and therapeutic applications of the B-chloroethyl amines and sulfides," *Science*, 103:409–415, 1946.

16. Goodman, L. S., Wintrobe, M. M., Dameshek, W., et al. "Nitrogen mustard therapy," *JAMA*, 132:126–132, 1946.

17. Karnofsky, D. A., Graef, I., and Smith, H. W. "Studies on the mechanism of action of the nitrogen and sulfur mustards in vivo," *Am. J. Pathol.*, 24:275–291, 1948.

18. Zubrod, C. G., Baker, C. G., Carrese, L. M., et al. "Part 1: history of the cancer chemotherapy program," *Cancer Chemother. Rep.*, 50:349–381, 1966.

19. Zubrod, C. G., Baker, C. G., Carrese, L. M., et al. "Summary of NCI appropriation in relation to grants, chemotherapy grants and chemotherapy contracts," *Cancer Chemother. Rep.*, 50:369, 1966.

20. Farber, S., Diamond, L. K., Mercer, R. D., et al. "Temporary remissions in acute leukemia in children produced by folic acid antagonist, 4-aminopteroyl-glutamic acid (aminopterin)," *N. Eng. J. Med.*, 238:787–793, 1948.

21. "Acute leukemia: present and future," *N. Eng. J. Med.*, editorial, 238:814–815, 1948.

22. "The lobby and the chair," *N. Eng. J. Med.*, editorial, 278:163–164, 1968.

23. Block, G. E., Jensen, E. V., and Polley, T. Z., Jr. "The prediction of hormonal dependency of mammary cancer," *Ann. Surg.*, 182:342–351, 1975.

24. Danten, R. J., Lipton, A., and Kendall, J. "Successful medical adrenalectomy with amino-glutethimide," *JAMA*, 230:1616–1665, 1974.

25. Frantz, A. G., Kleinberg, D. K., and Noel, G. L. "Studies on prolactin in man," in *Recent Progress in Hormone Research*, Astwood, E. B., ed. (New York: Academic Press, Inc., 1972), 28:527–571.

26. Kelley, R. M. "What chemotherapy should be used in metastatic breast cancer?" *Recent Results in Cancer Research*, 42:137–143, 1973.

27. Urtasun, R., Band, P., Chapman, J. D., et al. "Radiation and high-dose metronidazole in supratentorial glioblastomas," *Science*, 294:1365–1367, 1976.

28. Greenspan, E. M. *Clinical Cancer Chemotherapy* (New York: Raven Press, 1975).

29. Folkman, J. "The vascularization of tumors," *Sci. Am.*, 234:58–73, 1976.

30. Ackerman, L. V., and Rosai, J. *Surgical Pathology*, 5th ed. (St. Louis: C. V. Mosby Co., 1974).

31. Friedell, G. H., Betts, A., and Sommers, S. C. "The prognostic value of blood vessel invasion and lymphocytic infiltrates in breast carcinoma," *Cancer*, 18:164–166, 1965.

32. Ruiz, U., Babeu, S., Schwartz, M. S., et al. "Blood vessel invasion and lymph node metastasis: two factors affecting survival in breast cancer," *Surgery*, 73:185–190, 1973.

33. Fisher, B., Carbone, P., Economou, S. G., et al. "I-phenylalanine mustard (L-PAM) in the management of primary breast cancer: a report of early findings," *N. Eng. J. Med.*, 292:117–122, 1975.

34. Bonadonna, G., Brusamolino, E., Valagussa, P., et al. "Combination chemotherapy as an adjuvant treatment in operable breast cancer," *N. Eng. J. Med.*, 294:405–410, 1976.

35. Ravdin, R. G. Letter to Dr. Cope regarding the Breast Cancer Task Force, 1966.

36. Cope, O. Reply to letter from Ravdin regarding the Breast Cancer Task Force, 1966.

37. Holland, J. F. "Major advance in breast cancer therapy," *N. Eng. J. Med.*, 294:440, 1976.

38. Holland, J. F. "Breast cancer and chemotherapy," *Science*, 192:1062–1063, 1976.

39. Costanza, M. E. "The problem of breast cancer prophylaxis," *N. Eng. J. Med.*, 293:1095, 1975.
40. Culliton, B. J. "Breast cancer: reports of new therapy are greatly exaggerated," *Science*, 191:1029–1030, 1976.
41. Unsigned. "Unproven methods of cancer management: Hydrazine Sulfate," *CA: A Cancer Journal for Clinicians*, 26:108–110, 1976.
42. Culliton, B. J. "The trials of an apricot pit: 1973," *Science*, 182:1000–1003, 1973.
43. Eyerly, R. C. "Laetrile: focus on the facts," *CA: A Cancer Journal for Clinicians*, 26:50–54, 1976.
44. Unsigned. "Laetrile crackdown," *Time*, June 7, 1976.
45. Unsigned. "Unproven methods of cancer management: Krebiozen and Carcalon," *CA: A Cancer Journal for Clinicians*, 23:111–115, 1973.

Chapter 10

Immunotherapy — Immunity in the Prevention and Control of Breast Cancer   pages 127–142

1. Fitzpatrick, T. B., Pathak, M. A., and Brown, M. M. L. "Prevention of solar degeneration and sun-induced carcinoma of the skin," in *Melanoma and Skin Cancer*, McCarthy, W. H., ed. *Proc. Int. Cancer Conf.* (Sydney, New South Wales: V.C.N. Blight, Govt. printer, 1972).
2. Simpson, C. L., Hempelmann, L. H., and Fuller, L. M. "Neoplasia in children treated with x-rays in infancy for thymic enlargement," *Radiology*, 64:840–845, 1955.
3. Hugo, N. E. "The skin," Chapter 7, *Management of the Patient with Cancer*, 2nd ed., Nealon, T. F., ed. (Philadelphia: W. B. Saunders Co., 1976), p. 87.
4. Ibid., pp. 102–104, 1976.
5. Moore, F. D. "The gastrointestinal tract and the acute abdomen," in *Surgery*, Warren, R., ed. (Philadelphia: W. B. Saunders Co., 1963), p. 803.
6. Haagensen, C. D. *Diseases of the Breast*, 2nd ed. (Philadelphia: W. B. Saunders Co., 1971).
7. Allen, D. W., and Cole, P. "Viruses and human cancer," *N. Eng. J. Med.*, 286:70–82, 1972.
8. Bittner, J. J. "Possible relationship of the estrogenic hormones, genetic susceptibility, and milk influence in the production of mammary cancer in mice," *Cancer Res.*, 2:710, 1942.
9. Borden, E. C. "Viruses and breast cancer: implications of mouse and human studies," *The Johns Hopkins Medical Journal*, 134:66–76, 1974.
10. Breenan, M. J. "Murine and rat mammary tumors as models for

the immunological study of human breast cancer," *Cancer Res.*, 36:728–733, 1976.

11. Dulbecco, R. "From the molecular biology of oncogenic DNA viruses to cancer," *Science*, 192:437–440, 1976.

12. Glasser, R. J. *The Body Is the Hero* (New York: Random House, 1976).

13. Williams, G. Chapters 22–26, *Virus Hunters* (New York: Alfred A. Knopf, 1959).

14. Ibid., Chapter 27.

15. Alford, C., Hollinshead, A. C., and Herberman, R. B. "Delayed cutaneous hypersensitivity reactions to extracts of malignant and normal human breast cells," *Ann. Surg.*, 178:20–24, 1973.

16. Codington, J. F. Personal communication.

17. Coley, W. B. "The therapeutic value of the mixed toxins of the streptococcus of erysipelas and Bacillus prodigiosus in the treatment of inoperable malignant tumors, with a report of 160 cases," *Am. J. Med. Sci.*, 112:251–281, 1896.

18. Coley, W. B. "Spindle-celled sarcoma of the sternum successfully treated with the mixed toxins of erysipelas and Bacillus prodigiosus," *Ann. Surg.*, 47:805–807, 1908.

19. Nauts, H. C. Bibliography of reports concerning the clinical or experimental use of coley toxins (streptococcus pyogenes and serratia marcescens) 1893-1975 (New York: Cancer Research Institute Inc., 1975).

20. Everson, T. C., and Cole, W. H. "Spontaneous regression of cancer: preliminary report," *Ann. Surg.*, 144:366–383, 1956.

21. Ackerman, L. V., and Rosai, J. *Surgical Pathology*, 5th ed. (St. Louis: C. V. Mosby Co., 1974).

22. Crile, G., Jr. "Simplified treatment of cancer of the breast: early results of a clinical study," *Ann. Surg.*, 135:745–758, 1961.

23. Crile, G., Jr. "Possible role of uninvolved regional nodes in preventing metastasis from breast cancer," *Cancer*, 24:1283–1285, 1969.

24. Fisher, B., Wolmark, N., Coyle, J., et al. "Studies concerning the regional lymph node in cancer VIII: effect of two asynchronous tumor foci on lymph node cell cytotoxicity," *Cancer*, 26:521–527, 1975.

25. Girsch, M. S., Black, P. H., and Proffitt, M. R. "Immunosuppression and oncogenic virus infections," *Federations Proceedings*, 30:1852–1857, 1971.

26. Glasser, R. J. "Cancer," Chapter 16, in *The Body Is the Hero* (New York: Random House, 1976), pp. 206–225.

27. Prout, George. Personal communication, 1976.

28. Baltimore, D. "Viruses, polymerases, and cancer," *Science*, 192:632–636, 1976.

29. Temin, H. M. "The DNA provirus hypothesis," *Science*, 192:1075–1080, 1976.
30. Mathé, G., Amiel, J. L., Schwarzenberg, L., et al. "Active immunotherapy for acute lymphoblastic leukemia," *Lancet*, 1:697–699, 1969.
31. MacGregor, A. B., Falk, R. F., Landi, S., et al. "Oral Bacille Calmette Guérin immunostimulation in malignant melanoma," *Surg., Gynecol., and Obstet.*, 141:747–754, 1975.
32. Eilber, F. R., Morton, D. L., Holmes, E. C., et al. "Adjuvant immunotherapy with BCG in treatment of regional-lymph-node metastases from malignant melanoma," *N. Eng. J. Med.*, 294:237–240, 1976.
33. Monsaingeon, A. of the Groupe français d'immunologie et d'immunotherapie du cancer. Personal communication, 1975.
34. Gutterman, J. U., Blumenschein, G. R., Hortobagyi, G., et al. "Immunotherapy for breast cancer," *Breast*, 2:29–34, 1976.
35. Merson, M. H., Morris, G. K., Sack, D. A., et al. "Travelers' diarrhea in Mexico: a prospective study of physicians and family members attending a congress," *N. Eng. J. Med.*, 294:1299–1305, 1976.
36. Stein, M., Schiavi, R. C., and Camerino, M. "Influence of brain and behavior on the immune system," *Science*, 191:435–440, 1976.
37. Riley, V. "Mouse mammary tumors: alteration of incidence as apparent function of stress," *Science*, 189:465–467, 1975.

Chapter 11

Emotional Reactions to Cancer and the Mutilation of the Breast pages 143–157

I. Medical Literature:

1. Renneker, R., and Cutler, M. "Psychological problems of adjustment to cancer of the breast," *JAMA*, 148:833–838, 1952.
2. Bard, M. "The sequence of emotional reactions in radical mastectomy patients," *Public Health Reports*, 67:1144–1148, 1952.
3. Bard, M., and Sutherland, A. M. "Psychological impact of cancer and its treatment, IV: adaptation to radical mastectomy," *Cancer*, 4:656–672, 1955.
4. Eisenberg, H. S., and Goldenberg, I. S. "Measurement of quality of survival of breast cancer patients," in *Clinical Evaluation in Breast Cancer*, Hayward, J. L., and Bulbrook, R. D., eds. (New York: Academic Press, 1966), pp. 93–100.
5. Schottenfeld, D., and Robbins, G. F. "Quality of survival among

patients who have had radical mastectomy," *Cancer*, 26:650–654, 1970.

6. Markel, W. "The American Cancer Society's program for the rehabilitation of the breast cancer patient," *Cancer*, 28:1676–1678, 1971.

7. Crile, G., Jr. "The case for local excision of breast cancer in selected cases," *Lancet*, 2:7750–7752, 1972.

8. Holland, J. "Psychologic aspects of cancer," Chapter XVL-2, in *Cancer Medicine*, Holland, J. , and Frei, E. III, eds. (Philadelphia: Lea & Febiger, 1973).

9. Holleb, A. I. "Cancer therapy — the patient's decision?" *CA: A Cancer Journal for Clinicians*, 23:181, 1973.

10. Craig, T. J., Comstock, G. W., and Geiser, P. B. "The quality of survival in breast cancer: a case-control comparison," *Cancer*, 23:1451–1457, 1974.

11. Neeman, R. L., and Neeman, M. "Cancer prevention education for youth — a key for control of uterine and breast cancer," *J. Sch. Health*, 44:543–547, 1974.

12. Kent, S. "Coping with sexual identity crisis after mastectomy," *Geriatrics*, 30:145–146, 1975.

13. Greer, S., and Morris, T. "Psychological attributes of women who develop breast cancer: a controlled study," *J. Psychosom. Res.*, 19(2):147–153, 1975.

14. Schonfield, J. "Psychological and life-experience differences between Israeli women with benign and cancerous breast lesions," *J. Psychosom. Res.*, 19:(4)229–234, 1975.

15. Asken, M. J. "Psychoemotional aspects of mastectomy: a review of recent literature," *Am. J. Psychiatry*, 132:56–59, 1975.

16. Nadelson, C. "Post-mastectomy crisis," *Human Sexuality*, pp. 142, May 1975.

Nursing Literature:

17. Quint, J. C. "The impact of mastectomy," *Am. J. Nurs.*, 63:88–97, 1963.

18. Unsigned. "Women's attitudes regarding breast cancer," *Occup. Health Nurs.* (NY), 22(2):20–23, 1974.

19. Unsigned. "Fact and fantasy about breast cancer," *AORN Journal*, 19(4):845–850, 1974.

20. Akehurst, A. C. "Post-mastectomy morale," *Nursing Mirror*, 139(21):66, 1974.

21. Woods, N. F. "Psychologic aspects of breast cancer: review of the literature," *J. Obstet. , Gynecol. and Neonatal Nurs.*, 4(5):15–22, 1975.

22 Roberts, J. M. "Mastectomy — a patient's point of view," *Nurs. Times*, 71:1290–1291, 1975.

Psychology Literature:

23.   Lowe, C. M. "The self-concept: fact or antifact?" *Psychol. Bull.*, 58:325–336, 1961.

II. Plastic Surgical Reconstruction of
The Breast After Radical Mastectomy:

24.   Millard, D. R., Jr., Devine, J. Jr., and Warren, W. D. "Breast reconstruction: a plea for saving the uninvolved nipple," *Am. J. Surg.*, 122:763–764, 1971.

25.   Miller, S. H., and Graham, W. P. III. "Breast reconstruction after radical mastectomy," *Am. Fam. Physician*, 11:97–101, 1975.

III. Limited Excision in Recognition of Psychologic
Impact of Total Breast Removal:

26.   Mustakallio, S. "Treatment of breast cancer by tumour extirpation and roentgen therapy instead of radical operation," *Faculty Radiol.*, 6:23, 1954.

27.   Porritt, A. "Early carcinoma of the breast," *Br. J. Surg.*, 51:214, 1964.

28.   Peters, M. V. "Wedge resection and irradiation: an effective treatment in early breast cancer," *JAMA*, 200:144–145, 1967.

29.   Cope, O., Wang, C. A., Schulz, M., et al. "Breast cancer reconsidered: the rationale for radiation therapy without mastectomy," *Trans. N. Eng. Surg. Soc.*, October 1967.

30.   Cope, O. *Man, Mind and Medicine: The Doctor's Education* (Philadelphia: J. B. Lippincott Co., 1968).

31.   Cope, O. "Breast cancer: has the time come for a less mutilating treatment?" *Radcliffe Quarterly*, p. 6, June 1970.

32.   Cope, O. "Breast cancer: has the time come for a less mutliating treatment?" *Psychiatry Med.*, 2:263–269, 1971.

IV. Pathology and Others:

33.   Ackerman, L. V., and Rosai, J. "The pathology of tumors, Part Four: grading, staging and classification of neoplasms," *CA: A Cancer Journal for Clinicians*, 21:368, 1971.

34.   Long, J., and Castelman, B. In preparation.

35.   An account written by the same woman who described her thoughts about the mutilation of mastectomy in *Man, Mind and Medicine*, note 30, pp. 32–36.

36.   Stein, M., Schiavi, R. C., and Camerino, M. "Influence of brain and behavior on the immune system," *Science*, 191:435–440, 1976.

Chapter 12
The Shifting Emphasis in Diagnosis
and Treatment pages 158–174

The several issues and measures covered in this chapter have been discussed in detail in earlier chapters and full references were given. To avoid unnecessary duplication only those useful for emphasis and ready reference are repeated here.

1. Silverberg, B. S., and Holleb, A. I. "Major trends in cancer: 25-years survey," *CA: A Cancer Journal for Clinicians*, 25:2–21, 1975.
2. Third national cancer survey, incidence data, National Cancer Institute Monograph 41, Cutler, S. J., and Young, J. L., eds., March 1975.
3. Cutler, S. J., and Davesa, S. S. "Trends in cancer incidence and mortality in the U.S.A.," in Doll, R., and Vodopija, I. *Host Environment Interactions in the Etiology of Cancer in Man* (Lyon: International Agency for Research on Cancer, 1970).
4. Frantz, V. K., Pickren, J. W., Melcher, G. W., et al. "Incidence of chronic cystic disease in so-called 'normal breasts:' study based on 225 postmortem examinations," *Cancer*, 4:762–783, 1951.

Dr. Frantz and her colleagues found evidence of the fibrocystic disorder in 53 percent of women whose breasts were examined after death. Since the disorder may disappear spontaneously, with a pregnancy, or after the menopause, 53 percent is minimal. The true percentage is probably much higher. Earlier onset of menstruation and practice of birth control, among other factors, are presumably increasing its incidence.

5. Jones, C. H., Greening, W. P., Aavey, J. B., et al. "Thermography of the female breasts: a five-year study in relation to the detection and prognosis of cancer," *Br. J. Radiol.*, 48:532–538, 1975.
6. Kalisher, L., and Schaffer, D. L. "Xeromammography in early detection of breast cancer," *JAMA*, 234:60–63, 1975.
7. Kline, T. S., and Neal, H. S. "Needle aspiration detects breast cancer," *JAMA*, 227:15, 1974.
8. Furnival, C. M., Hughes, H. E., Hocking, M. A., et al. "Aspiration cytology in breast cancer: its relevance to diagnosis," *Lancet*, pp. 446–449, September 1975.
9. Ackerman, L. V., and Rosai, J. "The pathology of tumors, Part Four: grading, staging and classification of neoplasms," *CA: A Cancer Journal for Clinicians*, 21:368, 1971.
10. Ackerman, L. V., and Rosai, J. "Breast," Chapter 19, in *Surgical Pathology*, 5th ed. (St. Louis: C. V. Mosby Co., 1974).

11. Cope, O., Wang, C. A., Chu, A., et al. "Limited surgical excision as the basis of a comprehensive therapy for cancer of the breast," *Am. J. Surg.*, 131:400–407, 1976.

Chapter 13

Good Care, Now and in the Future   pages 175–188

1. Peters, V. M. "Wedge resection and irradiation: an effective treatment of early breast cancer," *JAMA*, 200:144–145, 1967.
2. Guttman, R. J. "Radiotherapy in the treatment of primary operable carcinoma of the breast with proved lymph node metastases: approach and results," *Am. J. Roentgenol. Radium Ther. and Nucl. Med.*, 89:58–63, 1963.
3. Cope, O. "Breast cancer: has the time come for a less mutilating treatment?" *Psychiatry Med.*, 2:263–269, 1971.
4. Montague, E. Personal communication, 1970.
5. Hershey, F. B., and Auer, A. I. Personal communication, 1973.
6. Nelson, A. J. III, and Montague, E. D. "Resectable localized breast cancer," *JAMA*, 231:189–191, 1975.
7. Prosnitz, L. R., and Goldenberg, I. S. "Irradiation for early breast Ca.," *Medical World News*, February 1975, p. 31.
8. Weber, E. T., and Hellman, S. "Radiation as primary treatment for local control of breast carcinoma," *JAMA*, 234:608–611, 1975.
9. Haagensen, C. D. *Diseases of the Breast*, 2nd ed. (Philadelphia: W. B. Saunders Co., 1971).
10. Costanza, M. E. "The problem of breast cancer prophylaxis," *N. Eng. J. Med.*, 293:1095, 1975.
11. Schulz, M. D. "The supervoltage story," Janeway Lecture, 1974, *Am. J. Roentgenol. Radium Ther. and Nucl. Med.* 124:541–559, 1975.
12. Sadowsky, N. L., Kalisher, L., White, G., et al. "Radiologic detection of breast cancer: review and recommendations," *N. Eng. J. Med.*, 294:370–373, 1976.
13. Unsigned. Medical News. "Critics, defenders express views about routine mammography," *JAMA*, 236:541–542, 1976.
14. Maloof, F. "Regulatory mechanisms of the pituitary-thyroid axis," Chapter 15, in *Pathophysiology: Altered Regulatory Mechanisms in Disease*, Frohlich, E. D., ed. (Philadelphia: J. B. Lippincott Co., 1972).
15. Albright, F., Smith, P. H., and Richardson, A. M. "Postmenopausal osteoporosis: its clinical features," *JAMA*, 116:2465, 1941.
16. Gordan, G. S., Picchi, J., and Roof, B. S. "Antifracture efficacy of long-term estrogens for osteoporosis," *Trans. Assoc. Amer. Phys.*, 86:326–332, 1973.

17. Gordan, G. S. "Preventing osteoporosis," *The Female Patient*, 1:45–49, 1976.
18. Gordan, G. S. Preface: "Symposium on Postmenopausal Osteoporosis, 10th International Congress of Gerontology," June 22–27, 1975, Jerusalem, Israel.
19. Rakoff, A. E. "Human neuroendocrinology: discussion, in *Advances in Neuroendocrinology*, Nalbandov, A. V., ed. (Urbana: University of Illinois Press, 1963), pp. 500–509.
20. Gloor, P. "Physiology of the limbic system," Chapter 3, in *Advances in Neurology*, Penry, J. K., and Daly, D. D., eds. (New York: Raven Press, 1975).

Figures A and B of the Lymphatic Drainage from a Cancer in the Right Breast

1. Rouvière, H. *Anatomie des lymphatiques de l'homme* (Paris: Masson, 1932).
2. Ibid., p. 157.
3. Handley, R.S., and Thackray, A.C. "Invasion of the internal mammary lymph glands in carcinoma of the breast." *Br. J. Cancer*, 1:15–20, 1974.
4. Turner-Warwick, R.T. "The lymphatics of the breast," *Br. J. Surg.*, 46:574–582, 1959.
5. Haagensen, C.D. "Anatomy of the Mammary Gland," Chapter 1 in *Diseases of the Breast*, 2nd ed. (Philadelphia: W. B. Saunders Co., 1971).

Index